PROFESSIONS, INFORMATION TECHNOLOGY AND MANAGEMENT IN HOSPITALS

For Ma and Pa

Professions, Information Technology and Management in Hospitals

MIKE DENT
School of Social Sciences
Staffordshire University

Avebury
Aldershot • Brookfield USA • Hong Kong • Singapore • Sydney

Published by
Avebury
Ashgate Publishing Limited
Gower House
Croft Road
Aldershot
Hants GU11 3HR
England

Ashgate Publishing Company
Old Post Road
Brookfield
Vermont 05036
USA

British Library Cataloguing in Publication data

Dent, Mike
Professions, information technology and management in hospitals
1. Hospitals - Administration - Data processing
I. Title
362.1'1'068

ISBN 1 85628 869 2

Library of Congress Catalog Card Number: 96-84597

Printed and bound by Athenaeum Press, Ltd.,
Gateshead, Tyne & Wear.

Contents

List of figures

List of tables

Acknowledgements

This book is the outcome of research and teaching carried out over a number of years. In the process I have been helped by a large number of people. First, there were the doctors, nurses, computer specialists and managers who gave of their time for the research. It is not possible to name them for that would breach the promises of confidentiality. The fact that they are anonymous, however, does not lessen my appreciation of their help and interest.

Different chapters benefited from advice, help and conversations with a range of people in particular Celia Davies, Tony Elger, Martin Parker Joel Richman and David Young who in their very different ways played a direct part in the development of the ideas contained in this book. There were also the students of the 'IT, Medicine and Care' modules at Manchester Metropolitan and Staffordshire Universities who have heard most of the contents of this book before. Ruth Green, David Cox, and Judy David worked with me on one of the case studies (reported in Chapter 3). I very much appreciate the help all have provided. None of them, however, can be held responsible for what I have written here.

Most of researches reported in this book have appeared in articles published earlier. In Chapter 3 the section on management strategies is derived from an article entitled 'Information technology and managerial strategies in the NHS: computer policies, organizational change and the labour process' that appeared in *Critical Perspectives on Accounting* (Volume 2, pp.331-60) (Dent, 1991) and appears here by kind permission of Acedemic Press. The later section on corporate systems draws on research that originally appeared in the chapter by Dent, Green, David and Cox (1992) in Loveridge and Starkey's edited collection *Continuity and Crisis in the National Health Service.* The discussion in Chapter 5 on medical audit is based on an article that appeared in The *Sociological Review* (Dent, 1993). Similarly, the case study in Chapter 6 is based on the article 'Organizations and change in renal work' that appeared in the *Sociology of Health and Illness* (Dent, 1990a) and most of Chapter 7 is based on an article entitled 'The new National Health Service: a case of postmodernism?' (Dent, 1995b) which was published in *Organization Studies* (Volume. 16, No. 5, pp.875-99) and appears here with the kind permission of the journal.

The research on which much of this book will be based has been funded from a number of sources. These were: The National Advisory Board (Programme 5, Project 38, 1988-91), ESRC (Reference GOO 230077, 1985), West Midlands Regional Health Authority (3 projects: 1984, 1985, 1986). To all these bodies I am most grateful.

Finally, Josie, Robin, Madeleine and Carol. Thanks.

Glossary of abbreviations

The abbreviations and acronyms are deciphered in the text. Nevetheless, this glossary may still be useful to the reader.

A&E	Accident and Emergency
ADNS	Assistant Director of Nursing Services
AHA	Area Health Authority
AI	Artificial Intelligence
AIM & TS	Association of Information Management and Technology Staff
ANT	Actor Network Theory
AT&T	American Telephone and Telegraph
BCS	British Computer Society
BJHC	British Journal of Healthcare Computing
BMA	British Medical Association
BMJ	British Medical Journal
CAPD	Continuous Ambulatory Peritoneal Dialysis
CASE	Computer-Aided Software Engineering
CAI	Computer-Aided Instruction
CAT	Computer-assisted tomography
CCPD	Continuous Cyclic Peritoneal Dialysis
CD-ROM	Compact Disc-Read Only Memory
CEPOD	Confidential Enquiry into Perioperative Deaths
CINAHL	Cumulative Index to Nursing and Allied Health Literature
CMMS	Case Mix Management System
COSTAR	COmputer STored Ambulatory Record
CT	Computerized Tomography
DHA	District Health Authority
DHSS	Department of Health and Social Security

DIP	Document Imaging Processing
DIS	District Information System
DP	Data Processing
DoH	Department of Health
DRG	Diagnosis Related Groups
DSS	Decision Support Systems
EDP	Electronic Data Processing
EPOR	Empirical Programme of Relativism
ESRF	End Stage Renal Failure
ETHICS	Effective Technical and Human Implementation of Computer-based Systems
FM	Facilities Management
FPC	Family Practitioner Committee
GDP	Gross Domestic Product
HCI	Human-Computer Interface
HIS	Health Information System
HISS	Hospital Information Support System
HN	Health Notice
HO	House Officer
HRG	Health Related Groups
IAV	Interactive Video Instruction
IBM	International Business Machines
ICD	International Classification of Diseases
ICL	International Computers Ltd
ICT	Information and Communications Technologies
IEEE	Institution of Electrical and Electronic Engineers.
IMG	Information Management Group.
IRC	Inter-Regional Consortium
IRC PAS	Inter-Regional Consortium - Patient Administration System
IRIS	Integrated Resource Information System
IT	Information Technology
JCC	Joint Consultants Committee
LAN	Local Area Network
LISP	LISt Processing (programming non-numeric information in artificial intelligence)
MEDICL	MEdical DIagnosis and Computer-aided Learning
MEDINFO	World Congress on Medical Informatics
MEDLINE	Medical Literature Analysis and Retrieval System On Line
MIS	Management Information System
MMS	Manpower Management System
MRC	Medical Research Council
MRI	Magnetic Resonance Imaging
MUMPS	Massachussetts General Hospital Multi-Progamming System
NAO	National Audit Office
NCR	National Cash Register
NMR	Nuclear Magnetic Resonance (scanner)

NMS or NMIS	Ward Nursing Management and Information System
NPHT	Nuffield Provincial Hospital Trust
O & M	Organizations and Methods engineering
OECD	Organization for Economic Cooperation and Development
PAC	Public Accounts Committee
PAS	Patient Administration System
pc	Personal computer
PET	Positron Emission Tomography
PICT	Programme on Information and Communication Technologies
POMR	Problem-Orientated Medical Records
PROMIS	Problem Orientated Medical Information System
PRP	Performance Related Pay
QA	Quality Assurance
RCC	Regional Computer Centre
RHA	Regional Health Authority
RMI	Resource Management Iniative
RSS	Regional Standard System
SAS	Standard Accounting System
SHO	Senior House Officer
SPS	Standard Payroll System
SPSS-X	Statistical Package for the Social Sciences (X is the mainframe version, PC+ is for pc use)
SSADM	Structured Systems Analysis and Design Method
SSM	Soft Systems Methodology
TORU	Technology and Organisations Research Unit.
UCE	University of Central England
UGM	Unit General Manager
UMIS	Unit Management Information System
VDU	Visual Display Unit
WAN	Wide Area Network
WIMPs	Windows, Icons, Mouse, Pull-down menus
WIMS	Works Information Management System
WISL	Wessex Information Systems Ltd
WMRHA	West Midlands Regional Health Autority
WORM	Write Once Read Many times
4GL	Fourth Generation (programming) Languages

1 Introduction

Introduction

This book is about the implications of information technology (IT) has for professional groups and their management within hospitals. The use of IT within hospitals has a surprisingly long history and dates back to well before the term IT came into common usage. It goes back at least 30 years to when batch 'punch-card' accounts systems were first introduced in the 1950s. Since that time computer technology has been applied to the whole spectrum of hospital activities as the systems became many times more powerful yet incredibly small compared to the forerunners. Nevertheless, as technological systems they belong to the same 'family'. It is important, however, not to overstate the continuity for there have been periods of dramatic change. In some ways the earliest generation of computers appear to be dinosaurs - a different and extinct species - rather than the direct antecedents of today's computer technology. The introduction of integrated circuits and transistor technology in the mid-1960s was a major breakthrough in creating reliable and economic database technology. It was, however, the introduction of the 'microchip' in the 1970s which provided the 'quantum leap' in the power and capacity of computers (Bylinsky, 1980; Saba and McCormick, 1986, pp.38-9) and made possible the flexible and ubiquitous mini- and micro-computers at the expense of the mainframe computer systems and the 'in-house' computer specialists who supported them. By the mid-1980s the technology had entered its 'fifth generation' with a particular focus on artificial intelligence (.i.Feigenbaum and McCorduck;, 1984; .i.Saba and McCormick;, 1986, pp.39-40). At the same time, however, the problems of interconnecting or 'networking' of computer systems were being resolved and extended to the fax machines and other communications technologies to create information and communications technologies (ICT). Computers have - since the 1950s - grown out of being just very rapid calculating machines and very useful filing systems (data-bases) to now it can be part of a multi-media integrated set of information and communication technologies.

Despite all these changes today's computer systems remain the direct descendants of the earlier 'punch-card' systems of the 1950s and part of the reason for this continuity is that computer systems (as with all technological artefacts) are socially *constructed*. Let me add at once this is not saying that technology is socially *created* but that technological systems emerge, develop and are sustained by social and organizational systems of people with different interests, concerns, power and influence. It is here that one finds the real disjunctions in the history of hospital computing. The most significant periods here were the mid 1960s and the 1980s and the period in-between was the heyday of NHS computing and the significance of these dates will be explained in subsequent chapters. It might be thought that the latter date is somehow related to the introduction of the 'internal market' but - whilst it did play its part - there was a prior one which was the desire of NHS management to wrest control of the systems from the technical specialists. This strategy was to have real consequences for the computer specialists employed within the NHS and it raised the question whether managers could now use the same or similar techniques to gain more direct control over the work of other professional groups within hospitals. This is a central issue examined within this book and in particular the implications the computer systems have had for the doctors, nurses as well as the computer specialists.

Before setting out the details of the argument in any further detail it will, first, be useful for me to describe the organization of the NHS as the changing organizational arrangements play an integral role in the overall argument. Then it will be possible to set out the general argument and the scope of the study. Next is a brief section of research methods and the chapter ends with a resume of the subsequent chapters.

The organizational context

From its beginning in 1948 until 1990 and the enactment of the *NHS and Community Care Act* the NHS organization was based on a highly bureaucratic and centralized structure with the Department of Health (DoH) at the centre and the health minister and Parliament at its apex (Ham, 1992; Ranade, 1994). This provided clear lines of administrative accountability and on the numbers of administrative staff required to run the service. The service was based on 14 regional health authorities (RHAs) for England who oversaw the work of the 192 district health authorities (DHAs) who, in turn, were responsible for the organization of the hospitals in their locality. Hospital administration was at the very bottom of this hierarchy. Doctors, on the other hand, were not.

Despite the strong centralized structure the balance of power within the service has not necessarily favoured the Department of Health. Doctors in Western medicine generally have long enjoyed a particular form of authority and occupational power which Freidson (1970) has labelled medical dominance. With the establishment of the NHS medical dominance became particularly influential in the management of hospitals and on matters of day-to-day operations the government were content to leave de facto control to the doctors. This did not mean, however, that there were not areas of conflict between state and the profession. One issue of long-standing government concern was the cost of medicine. While Parliament allocated the resources it was the doctors who principally decided how the monies were spent. Something like 80 per cent of all health costs were generated by doctors' medical decisions (Schroeder, 1980). In the wake of the Resource Management Initiative doctors do appear to becoming more cost-conscious. Nevertheless, they still enjoy clinical autonomy and collegiate solidarity which enables them to still avoid complying with policies they do not agree with (e.g. Ham, 1992, pp.177-80; Dent, 1993).

The basic assumption behind the setting up of the NHS in 1948 was that this new 'free at point of delivery' service would systematically clear up a backlog of ill health known to exist in the community (Ham, 1992, p.38). Thus the health service was a modernist project in itself designed to free the people from the burden of illness and disease. The premise, however, turned out to be false and the hospital service grew rather than shrank in size and complexity. By the 1970s the 'apparently inexorably increasing costs of all Western health services coincided with the end of an "era of optimism" about the contribution of high technology scientific medicine was making to health' (Elston, 1991, p.68). Even so acute hospitals continue to be dependent on expensive high-technology in part because control and evaluation of such systems are insufficiently rigorous (Ranade, 1994, p.39). Another perhaps more central challenge to the health service has been the 'greying' demography of UK society. As in other Western societies Britain too has an ageing population and older people require more health service support than their younger counterparts although, for the most part, they do not require high technology treatment (ibid., pp.33-6).

In consequence, the cost of the NHS has continued to rise and become a cause of concern for government. This was the case even though the UK spent proportionally less than any other Western European country. According to OECD data the UK spent 6.2 per cent of its Gross Domestic Product (GDP) on health as compared to 8.8 per cent by France, 8.1 per cent by Germany and 7.7 per cent by Italy (Schieber et al., 1992, p.4). Even so the British government felt impelled to introduced the 'internal market' into the NHS organization as a means of controlling costs and increasing the efficiency of the service. This was contained in the *NHS and Community Care Act* (1990) that also incorporated the other changes contained in the White Paper *Working for Patients* (1989). The essential difference, is that now hospitals are no longer administratively part of a monolithic NHS but, ostensibly, independent competitive contractors to the health authorities and fundholding general practitioners (e.g. Ranade, 1994, pp.65-81).

The general argument

The changes that NHS hospitals have undergone over the last 10 years have in important part been predicated on sophisticated computer networks. In principle this has been in order for hospital managers to be able to cope with the increased complexity entailed in the new systems of resource management and the internal market. These new organizational systems have also entailed a new configuration of control and influence as between managers, doctors, nurses and computer specialists. Health professions have now to be far more managerially responsible for their own activities than previously. Whether this means they are now subject to over-arching IT control systems is one of the questions to be addressed.

IT, and especially the rhetoric surrounding the subject, has played an important component in the restructuring of the NHS. In the early days of healthcare computing developments were very much 'technology-led' now it is very much 'information-led'. The was a change-over from one to the other which occurred during the 1980s and had important consequences for everyone involved in healthcare computing. No longer was it thought that IT would - of itself - bring benefits in wondrous if ill-defined ways. Instead, the technology was to be tamed and become the instrument of management. IT networks, case-mix management systems (CMMS) and Hospital Information Support Systems (HISS) (plus all the other IT components of health information systems) are now intended to provide the information necessary for the efficient and cost effective running of the service. Moreover, to ensure that the computer systems were the servants of management and not just a source of confusion, the work of the computer specialists was 'contracted out' and market competition relied upon to ensure managers were no longer victims of the computer gobbledygook. All these matters are the concern of the book within which I pursue two inter-related aims: first, to describe and analyze the development of IT within NHS hospitals and second, to examine the inter-relations between computer use and work processes of health professions and hospital management. The book is not primarily concerned with the technicalities of computing or computer systems.

In analyzing the interconnections between the rise of IT and the changing configuration of professional work and managerial relations the main argument draws on three main discourses: labour process, actor network and post-bureaucratic organizational theories. These form the basis of the proposition that healthcare computing and IT systems are predominantly social constructions. Whilst, there are several caveats that will need to be made to this statement the central point remains and that is healthcare computing and IT systems are more the outcome of organizational politics and the demands of hospital work than the secular advance of computer technology and science.

The scope of the study

This book covers healthcare computing in NHS acute hospitals within England and Wales. It does not cover hospitals in Scotland and Northern Ireland as there are important differences in the history and organization of hospital computing within. Non-acute hospitals have been ignored because IT has played less of a role there than in the acute sector. The main reason for focusing solely on the hospital sector (in England and Wales) is that it is a central component in the configuration of health care services and for that alone warrants attention. Moreover, some acute hospitals were among the first to experiment with computer systems and, later, all hospitals within the new 'internal market' have had to introduce new systems to support resource management and contracting arrangements. The focus, however, is not exclusively on the NHS for I do draw extensively on evidence from other parts of the world, especially the USA where many of the ideas and systems have first been tried.

A long established objective of many within the NHS has been to establish an integrated set of computer-based information systems to improve the management and delivery of hospital services and patient care. The IT in the title corresponds closely to another term often used, namely, 'healthcare computing' as, for example, in the title of 'The British Journal of Healthcare Computing and Information Management'. This technology does not include the hospital equipment used for investigations and therapies such as CAT or NMR 'scanners', haemo-dialysis machines and the like. IT systems will draw data from these sources and, increasingly, the equipment will be closely integrated within hospitals' IT networks. Nevertheless, the focus here is on the automation of the information and data not the procedures. While it is true that the boundary between the two is not always clear-cut a distinction can easily be made. IT is the computer-support for information and decision-making systems not the automated control of the machines. The decision-making may relate directly to the work of doctors and nurses or feed into wider information systems that are intended to underpin a hospital's management information system. In this book I will use the terms IT in the general sense of computer-based information systems and restrict the use of healthcare computing to computerized clinical activities and medical records. Another term in common use, is 'computer-based' and this will also be used from time to time as, for example, in the case of 'computer-based medical records systems'. Other terms, such as knowledge-based and artificial intelligence will be explained within the appropriate chapter as will the current 'acronyms and abbreviations such as HISS (Hospital Information Support Systems) and CMMS (Case Mix Management System).

Having established the boundaries to the subject matter it is now appropriate to delineate the analytical framework adopted. It may best be described as a sociology of organizations approach which is a 'mezo' level analysis focusing here on the organization of hospitals. There is impressionistically a certain attraction to this kind of configurational approach for tend to live out much of our lives within organizations: most of us were born in hospitals, went to school and college and work in offices and factories as well as shop in super-markets. We experienced these organizations as real - we walked through doors to get into and out of the buildings that housed them - yet they are also abstract constructs. Organizations are also to be understood as systems, cultures, processes, transactions and so on (e.g. Burrell and Morgan, 1979; Morgan, 1986; Hassard and Pym, 1990). It is not only in the world of theory, however, that organizations have become abstractions. This has happened in the 'real world', as it were, too. For many the organization is now a very nebulous phenomenon made up of contractually linked networks of actors (Powell, 1991). A practical example of this development is the NHS that has been radically altered with the introduction of the 'internal market'. It is no longer an integrated hierarchy but a collection of separate units contracted to deliver health care services at a given price and quality. In this new world of contingent relations it may be only the IT networks that provide the continuity and temporal existence of the NHS although, as will be made clear in later chapters, such a conclusion would be premature.

Research methods

This book is largely based on my own researches on the NHS since the early 1980s and has provided the case studies included in all the substantive chapters. In Chapters 3 (Computers, management and the state) and 4 (Computer Specialists and the emergence of the 'hybrid') these are based on literature reviews and a range of interviews and conversations with NHS computer specialists, regional managers and, early on in the research, members from the health marketing divisions of ICL, IBM and NCR. An important part of the research rationale, particular in relation to the journal searches, was to find and present documentary corroboration for the accounts given or, alternatively, provide counter-factual evidence. Here I made much use of The British Journal of Healthcare Computing (BJHC).

Chapters 5 to 7 each includes a qualitative case study and there is also a similar study contained within Chapter 3. The researches that underpin these case studies were based on semi-structured interviews, observations, informal conversations and internal documentation (reports, minutes, etc.). The research strategy adopted was a 'multiple strategic' one (Burgess, 1984) which, whilst being very similar to 'triangulation' (Denzin, 1978) in its terms of methods used is, in epistemological terms, quite different (Burgess, 1984, pp.144-6). The key difference between the two is that 'triangulation' is intended to provide objective findings, whilst the 'multiple strategic' approach is designed to provide an integrated, richly textured and comprehensive account (Burgess, 1984, p.146). Another way of expressing the same point would be to say that the 'multiple strategic' approach is a systematic attempt to *understand* the situation whereas 'triangulation' is designed on the assumption it can *prove* something in a positivistic way (Silverman, 1985, p.105).

All the case studies, except the one in Chapter 3, were based on studies covering periods of between 12 months to two years. The study of corporate systems in Chapter 3 is based on the same basic methodology as the others but only covered a 4 month period (in 1986) (Dent et al., 1992). All are concerned with peoples' responses to changes in their work either because of the introduction of new computer systems or organizational rearrangements or both. Typically the studies comprised of a 3-4 month round of interviews and observations (mainly meetings) on a weekly/fortnightly basis supplemented by an accumulation of 'in-house' documents on the subject. There then followed a break of several months before a second round of interviews and observations and literature search and in some cases there were further research rounds. This mode of working meant I was able to gain much more of a temporal (e.g. Hammersley and Atkinson, 1995, pp.225-6) and processual (Elger, 1975) perspective than would be possible from a 'before' and 'after' study for hospital computer systems cannot be treated just as independent variables 'injected' into an organization. Rather they are the outcome of social and organizational networks into which they may well become absorbed.

It is because of the complexity of social settings (including hospitals) that qualitative research needs to be theoretically based. Only by being so can it have any claim to validity different from journalism or travellers tales. Field research data has to be analyzed within a coherent and defensible theoretical framework that, firstly, provides a common set of reference points between studies and, second, is itself subject to interrogation by the researcher in light of the empirical data (and the contingent quality of that data). This is an important component of reflexivity in the sense that the 'theory' may be constantly subject to amendment, elaboration and even change. This is not quite the same as 'grounded theory' (Glaser and Strauss, 1967) because the researcher here enters the field with a basic organizing framework. Even so, there is no 'one best theory' (despite the heat involved in some academic debates) and it is quite feasible to analyze the same data drawing on different sociological paradigms (Burrell and Morgan, 1979; Hassard, 1990, pp.221-2; 1992). The subsequent analysis will emphasize different aspects of the subject matter under study and the ethical and political implications may be very different (Parker, 1993, pp.209-11). This is why the researcher has to reflexively monitor her/his own values and interests (e.g. Hammersley and Atkinson, 1995, pp.16-17). Certainly that is what I tried to do in the researches reported in this book.

The plan of the book

The structure of the book is as follows. Following this introduction is the 'theory' chapter which sets out the framework for the sociological analysis of healthcare computing. Some readers, however, may wish to 'skip' this and go straight for the topics of their particular interest. They should have little difficulty in doing so as each chapter is written so that it may be read independently. At the same time, however, the chapters are assembled in such a way they each contribute to the overall argument. Chapter 3 sets the historical and organizational context of health care computing within the NHS. It includes a discussion of the different and changing schema's of IT growth and the politics and processes behind the shift from the earlier technologically-led strategies to the information-led strategies that followed the Griffith's reforms. This provides the basis for the discussions in the following chapters of specific profession's adoption and uses of computer systems. Thus Chapters 4 to 6 discuss healthcare computing in relation to the work of computer specialists, doctors and nurses. The story of the changing fortunes of computer specialists is discussed in Chapter 4 which also covers the issues of professionalism and professionalization as well as the putative emergence of the 'IT dependent' hospital and computer 'hybrids' (Earl, 1989; Rose, 1991) and the emergence of information management.

Hospital doctors are the subject of Chapter 5. This professional group has had an even greater influence the 'shape' of healthcare computing than the computer specialists if, for no other reason, they have enjoyed a position of medical dominance (Freidson, 1970) within the hospital division of labour. The question of artificial intelligence is discussed and examples of knowledge-based systems are examined. Another important theme here is the automation of clinic notes and medical records, the implications this may have for medical work and doctors' responses to such developments. The discussion is supported by a case study of the introduction of a system into a midlands hospital. The chapter ends with a discussion of the medical audit and its role within the new NHS management systems.

Unlike the computer specialists and hospital doctors the nurses (Chapter 6) appear to have had little influence on the shaping of healthcare computing. Similarly, IT has had very limited impact on nursing work until relatively recently. Early nursing systems tended to concentrate on staffing and workloads this has now extended to include nursing records, care plans and ward management. Much of the nurses' practical involvement with IT systems, however, has been on behalf of others, inputting data for doctors and managers rather than themselves. A central issue for nursing is the possible conflict between technical rationality (of the new IT systems) and the emotional labour (Hochschild, 1983) and/or sentimental work (Strauss, et al., 1982, 1985). This is discussed in a case study which compares the responses of the nurses at two renal units to the introduction of a new computer system.

Chapter 7 is concerned with the new organizational arrangements and exploring how best to understand the ways in which management functions are now distributed among nurses and doctors as well as the hospital managers. The chapter starts with a review of the main 'post-bureaucratic' organizational theories (post-Fordism and post-modernism) as well as the populist 'McDonaldization' thesis. The discussion pays particular attention to the introduction of the 'internal market' and the intended role for IT. The case study explores these changes as they are experienced at the local level. In the final chapter current developments in data imaging processing, multi-media clinical work stations and related technologies are looked at in terms of their potential to overcome user-resistance and undermine the variant of social constructionist argument set out in this book. I then go on to summarise the themes and issues raised and conclude as I began that computer technology has played an ambivalent role in the restructuring of NHS hospitals and far more important in the construction of the IT systems has been the role played by the politics of professionalism.

2 The social 'shaping' of healthcare computing

Introduction

Hospitals have provided the setting for innovation in computer systems and technology since their first introduction and they have played an integral part in the policy and organizational changes that have occurred since. This role has, however, been a complex one for it has probably created as many dilemmas for those involved as it has solutions. This ambivalence serves as a central theme of this book and will be explored further in the subsequent chapters. Hospitals are clearly not the only setting for the development of these technologies although it has played a central role in certain areas, notably artificial intelligence (AI) (Chapter 5). More generally information technology (IT) (especially the micro-electronic components) can be viewed as one of the key 'heartland' technologies (McLoughlin and Clark, 1994, p.13) that are expected to play a central role the renaissance of industry and the economy. A distinctive characteristic of this particular technology is that it is represents a *process* rather than *product* innovation for its importance lies in its capacity to facilitate other innovations in 'firms and industries and the emergence of new forms of management, organization and economic activity' (ibid., p.13) rather than what they are in themselves. For instance this Macintosh LC III I am using at the moment is enabling me to write this book directly into camera-ready copy without the need or help of typists, print-setters and others. The introduction of the personal computer also had implications for the employment prospects and skills of computer specialists which is discussed in Chapter 4. The main point here, however, is that the micro-electronics base to this machine has made it very different to the technology of the author - the type-writer - and of a wide range of other occupations as well including secretaries, journalists and university lecturers. Networked together these machines can provide the information systems support for new forms of management. Micro-electronic process technologies have radically increased the processing power, speed, reliability and flexibility of computer and information systems whilst decreasing both their cost and size' (ibid., p.15).

One might, in light of all this evidence, be justifiably in awe of the scientists, engineers and technical specialists who - with prescience - invented and developed this world of micro-electronics wizardry. As stated, however, this interpretation privileges too much the technology in assuming that the new technology somehow preceded the demand for it. The relationship between invention, development and diffusion of new technologies is a complex one (ibid., pp.8-33) and one crucial component so far ignored is the process of social 'shaping' which plays a significant role in determining how they will, or will not, develop and be used. This is the subject of this chapter as it pertains to healthcare computing systems.

This chapter organized in the following way. It starts with a critical review of the healthcare computing literature before broadening out to include consideration of the wider sociological and organizational literature. It is at this stage I introduce labour process and social constructionist theories which are discussed in light of some aspects of Foucault's theory on power. My purpose is to construct a theoretical framework within which it is possible to explain how social, organizational and political processes have 'shaped' the design, use and effectiveness of information technology in healthcare organizations.

Healthcare computing literature

There exists a body of journals and conference proceedings that constitute a recognisable healthcare computing literature. Much of this consists of the conference papers and research reports that find their way into the publications of MEDINFO (Medical Informatics) and IEEE proceedings as well articles on computing found in medical and nursing journals and the like. In the UK the British Journal of Healthcare Computing & Information Management (BJHC & IM) has been an important source of information on IT developments both within the pages of the journal and the proceedings of its annual conference. The professional bodies also publish articles on computing within the pages of their journals intermittently. The review of this literature offered here represents a survey only and is not definitive. Much of this literature tends to be either of an ephemeral nature or too specific for the present purpose. Nevertheless, within this literature the following three basic theoretical models are clearly discernible:

1. Systems
2. Human Factor
3. Diffusionist

Each of these models will be examined in turn and their contribution to our understanding of the social and organizational impact of healthcare computing assessed. This will then lay the basis for the broader theoretical discussion in the second half of the chapter.

Systems models

This model plays a paradigmatic role for both health professionals and computer personnel. Both groups treat the systems model as a basis for action. Not for them the uncertainties of reification or objectivity expressed by sociologists (Silverman, 1970; 1994; Elger, 1975; Brown, 1992, pp. 82-3) rather their approaches implicitly assumes the possibility of a perfectable analysis or diagnosis which led Boguslaw (1965) to refer to the systems designers, programmers and engineers, if not the doctors, as the 'new utopians'. Both medicine and systems analysis, for instance, are heavily dependant upon assumptions of closed and partially closed systems (Silverman, 1970, pp.32-5). Medical students are trained to develop their diagnostic skills by assuming the patient is a combination of discrete systems (e.g. circulatory, respiratory, urinary, reproductive and even social). The practice of hospital medicine may vary considerably from the medical school model, but doctors rarely repudiate the model altogether (see Chapter 5). Computer and systems personnel are even more firmly rooted in the systems universe (Checkland, 1981; Checkland and Scholes, 1990, pp.18-20). This commitment has very practical consequences for the acceptability of computer systems. Systems analysts commonly equate acceptability to a set of previously agreed criteria between themselves and the 'users'. The criteria demarcate the boundaries of responsibilities for the systems personnel and once met defines the job as satisfactorily completed (see Chapter 4). This is the case whether or not the users are content with the new system. This formalism, for that is what it appears to be, is part of a broader problem with the too ready acceptance of the systems paradigm. I refer here to the formal assumption that there is only one organizational reality. Informally, systems analysts and designers know that there are other realities captured for instance in office gossip or the yellow 'post-it' reminders stuck all over the computer terminal. These, however, are treated as residual categories that may impinge on the efficiency of the system but are not an integral part of it.

Systems theory has perhaps been most trenchantly criticized by Burns (Brown, 1992, p. 81). The assumption that there is only one level of organizational reality - which Burns (1969, pp.232-49) referred to as the working system - is inadequate. An organization, according to Burns (ibid., p.241), can be viewed as comprising of three inter-related systems, (i) the working organization, (ii) the political system, and (iii) the career structure and the relationship between them is not one of potential technical integration but 'must be a moral ordering' (ibid., p.248) relating to the wider society. Silverman (1970, p.40) argued similarly that these arrangements ('systems') are to be best understood as 'a series of games, each with its own meanings and standards of expected behaviour'. What might be desirable by senior management may not be attainable or if attainable not experienced as positively by those who have to work with the systems. Integrated systems may have more in common with surveillance than harmonious relationships. A point that is taken up later in this chapter under the sub-head: *Strategy and Disciplinary Power*: The work of the Brunel Health Services Organizational Research Unit provides a particularly useful example of the approach from within the healthcare literature.

In both 'Hospital Organization' (Rowbottom et al., 1973) and 'Health Services' (Jaques et al., 1978) a systems model is used based on Jaques (1951). This originated out of the classic Glacier Metals study (Clegg and Dunkerley, 1980, p.204) and evolved for use in a health service context by Rowbottom (1977). Within this model the clinical autonomy of hospital doctors, for example, is not viewed as the outcome of the doctor's 'dignity, status and power' (Tolliday, 1978, p.42). Instead it is functionally defined as necessary for maintenance of patient trust and clinical confidentiality within the doctor-patient relationship. Moreover, it is subject to systematic monitoring arrangements, 'to ensure that clinicians keep within the law, binding professional standards, and NHS policy and resource limits ...' (ibid., p.41). This functional interpretation is over simplistic, for clinical autonomy is a crucial element of the autonomy enjoyed by doctors independent of the organizational imperatives of the health service (Freidson, 1970, p.45).

The Human Factor approach

The Human Factor approach is rooted in applied psychology and its adherents argue that, in the case of computers, it is necessary to design human acceptability into the very systems themselves. The approach is now commonly referred to as 'Human Computer Interaction' (HCI) by computer professionals. There is an HCI specialist group within the British Computer Society (BCS) and it forms an important component of accredited education and training programmes. This approach has its roots in the industrial psychology of C. S. Myers and others associated with the National Institute of Industrial Psychology whose central concerns related to practical questions of ergonomics and the improvement of the psychological well-being of workers at work (Rose, 1988, pp.61-100). In this earlier form '(p)sychology and biology were still intimately linked' (Rose, 1988, p.63) this is no longer the case with the HCI approach. Now it is cognitive psychology (e.g. Schneiderman, 1987) that provides the predominant theoretical underpinning although its general approach is a practical user-centred one (e.g. Rector, et al., 1988, pp.213-15).

Within the specific area of medical computing it has been in the area of medical decision-making that cognitive psychology would appear to have contributed most. In this country, it has been the MRC Social and Applied Psychology Unit at the University of Sheffield that has been the consistent champion of the human factor approach as the basis of good computer systems design and their acceptability. In the 1970s this work was associated with Fox (1977, pp.669-86; 1979, pp.425-31) and from the 1980s it was Fitter, with others, who been researching and writing on the subject (e.g. Fitter and Sime, 1980; Fitter and Cruikshank, 1983). But while it was these researchers who 'raise[d] human factors issues specific to the medical consultation environment' in their work (Fitter and Cruikshank, 1983, p.81) their studies led them to the view that HCI design needed to be based on more than the specific dialogues, task analysis, work station design, etc. because of the 'additional complexities of the three way interaction[s] (doctor, computer, patient) in a sensitive environment' (ibid., p.91). This led them to explore conversational analysis, in association with the sociologist Heath (ibid.). This is a development that may reflect a growing interest in the contribution that sociological analysis (of a particular kind) might make or, alternatively, reflect the researchers' recognition of the limitations of psychology. Whichever it was it was rooted in pragmatic rather than epistemological considerations.

Diffusionist models

Many commentators and analysts, particularly in the USA, have turned to diffusion theory[1] for an explanation of healthcare computing developments (Greer, 1977, 1981; Lindberg, 1979; Kaplan, 1982; Jay and Anderson, 1982, Anderson and Jay, 1983). Rogers (1962; Rogers and Shoemaker, 1971) based his now classic model on Merton's classification 'localites' or 'cosmopolites' to identify those most likely to be susceptible to new ideas and innovations and argued that, following Coleman et al. (1966), the persons who adopted the innovations acted as the opinion leaders among their peer groups. The study of Coleman et al (1966) is particularly relevant here for it concerns medical innovation, specifically the process by which doctors came to adopt new drugs in their clinics. The researchers found that it was the younger, better educated, more competent and geographically mobile 'cosmopolite' doctors who were the first to be aware of new drugs, and then to use them. Anderson and Jay (1983, pp.45-52) came to parallel conclusions in their later study computer utilization in clinical practice. The authors concluded that their study, 'demonstrate(d) the importance of peer influences ... in the introduction of computer technology' (ibid., p.51). This, however, was only a small-scale study of a group of physicians in one US hospital. The findings can only be taken as indicative rather than conclusive evidence.

Coleman et al. (1966) and Anderson and Jay (1983) assumed that opinion leaders would always equate the new with the desirable and demonstrate a 'cosmopolite' habit of promoting innovation. This assumption, however, is not necessarily warranted, for as Greer (1977, p.509) has pointed out:

> [O]pinion leaders may use their influence to speed up or slow down the diffusion process. Similarly, cosmopolites may, in perfect accord with standards of their reference groups, distrust proposed innovation.

But, she goes on to argue, even if the link between innovation, opinion leaders and cosmopolitanism matched the requirements of the diffusion model the theory could not adequately explain the organizational adoption of innovation, at least, not without shifting the focus of analysis away from the network of relations between opinion leaders and colleagues 'toward organizational and political theory' (ibid., p.506) which could then account for the negotiation of the organizational policies relating to innovation based on interests, resources and strategies (ibid) - a model that has much in common with Pettigrew's early analysis of organizational decision-making (1973a) and with the more recent developments in actor networks and social construction of technology models (see below).

Both Pettigrew (1972, 1973a) and Greer (1977) argue that diffusion theory requires further elaboration and recognition be given to the interplay of communications and power:

> [D]ecision makers negotiate policies and determine the interests, resources and strategies which they bring to the decision process. (Greer, 1977, p.506)

Greer, however, did not go beyond pointing to the desirability of a broad based model that would overcome the limitations of diffusion theory (ibid., p.529). Pettigrew, on the other hand, did develop a detailed model of the missing component from the classic diffusionist model, namely the decision processes (concerning innovation). His solution was to combine the concept of 'gatekeeper' with the assumption that communication systems within organizations were themselves power systems (1972, p.188). This model parallels the social constructionist approach (especially Pinch and Bijker, 1984, 1987), to be discussed later, in identifying social processes (i.e. organizational politics) that 'shape' the form and application of technological systems.

Healthcare computing literature and theory: an assessment

In broad terms, systems, human factor and diffusionist approaches are not to be thought of as wholly discrete, or mutually exclusive. They have commonly been used to account for the state of development and acceptability of computing in healthcare. For the most part the concern of researchers and commentators has been to explain the apparent resistance of health professionals to the use of computers. 'Human factors' research has concentrated on technical issues, including cognitive aspects of screen designs and ergonomics, but has ignored the wider but no less relevant issues of organizational and occupational power relations. Moreover, resistance may reflect the inappropriateness of the computer system to the work process (Kaplan, 1982; Young, 1984a) and not the psychological predisposition of the users, nor the proximity of innovative colleagues. In order to address all these issues it is necessary to look beyond the 'one dimensionality' of systems models, the narrowly constrained focus of human factors and develop further the insights of the diffusionist approach beyond its early optimistic and over-simple assumption that innovation is always a good thing. In order to develop such an alternative it is useful to examine two alternative approaches. First, labour process theory which, despite limitations, can help us better understand the interplay between the professional and managerial strategies involved. Secondly, social constructionist approaches to technology which concentrate on technological artefacts and systems and their diffusion.

Labour process and the social construction of technological systems [2]

Labour process theory and research have made a significant contribution to the study of new technology in the workplace (e.g. Noble, 1979, 1985; Wilkinson, 1983). Although the basic model as set out by Braverman (1974) does present problems with its over simplistic assumptions relating to the introduction of new technologies (e.g. Wilkinson, 1983, pp.12-16; Child, 1985, pp.107-41). Moreover, the original model was unable to account directly for technological change within public sector organizations. As it happens this does not of itself create an insurmountable problem. Indeed, labour process analysis has an important role in this book in clarifying the relationship between professions and the state. The second approach, social construction of technological systems, has very different origins for it emerged from the sociology of science and is pre-occupied with the processes by which technological artefacts become accepted. There are two distinct but overlapping strands in the work of this school: social constructionism and actor networks. The former is particularly associated with the work of Pinch and Bijker (1984; 1987) and emphasizes the social processes involved in the negotiated acceptance of a technological artefact or system. The latter, actor network theory, combine humans and non-humans into hybrid networks in which translation is the process (to be described later in this chapter) by which artefacts and systems come into social existence (Callon, 1986, 1987; Latour, 1993). My interest in these two discrete models (labour process and social constructionism) relate to their potential to account for the various strategies and practices relating to healthcare computer systems and their diffusion within the NHS hospital service. This is not to deny that there are problems of compatibility between the two approaches. The social constructionists embrace a general relativism and avoid any 'privileging' in the 'seamless web' of technology (Bijker et al., 1987, p.3) while labour process theory, by contrast, is committed to an ultimately economistic paradigm (Thompson, 1990, pp.99-101). The problem of incompatibility is capable of resolution, however, if the key ideas are viewed through a Foucauldian lens.

The labour process and the problems with professionals and technology

Labour process analysis, in its modern form, was the creation of Braverman (1974). Prior to the publication of his *Labor and Monopoly Capital* there had been 'no continuing body of work in the Marxist tradition dealing with the capitalist mode of production in the manner in which Marx treated it in the first volume of Capital' (Braverman, 1974, p.9). Braverman's re-focusing of academic attention directly onto work processes, practices and relations set the agenda for industrial sociology, industrial relations and organizational theory for the 1970s and 1980s. Nevertheless, it was clear from the beginning that Braverman's uni-dimensional approach with its reliance on scientific management as the sole managerial strategy for labour control and basis for accumulation was too deterministic. Research and historical evidence indicated that the degradation of labour was not as inescapable as he supposed (Child, 1985; Knights and Willmott, 1990, pp.10-12). This, however, has led not to a rejection of his work but to its reappraisal. Despite its weaknesses its focus on the organization and control of work both within production and the wider economic and social relations are too important to ignore. Instead the Braverman model has become a basis on which to elaborate. Friedman (1977, p.100), as one important early contributor, developed the distinction between *direct control* and *responsible autonomy*; thus contrasting two main types of managerial strategies, one the logic of scientific management the other that of the socio-technicism of the Tavistock Institute. Another early revisionist was Edwards (1979, pp.177-83) who extended Braverman's model by including three types of labour markets and an equal number of management control strategies. This was presented as a matrix of nine control strategies that contrasts considerably with Braverman's one of degradation and deskilling. Doctors and nurses, for example, are are identified as occupying the 'independent primary [labour] market' (ibid., pp. 174-7) which provides them with stable employment, job security, career progression and relatively high pay'. They are also identifiable as being under 'bureaucratic control' within the NHS which, together with their labour market position, corresponds closely with the notion of *responsible autonomy*. Burawoy (1979), by contrast, adopted a games model approach to labour process as an attempt to explain the generally high level of worker compliance. All these modifications can be seen as attempts to remain within a broadly integrated Marxist political economy where the relations between management and worker on the shopfloor are a microcosm of the wider political economy.

While labour process discourse is wide ranging it, nevertheless, has some serious limitations. Firstly, it has concentrated on manufacturing and service sector work within the private sector. Secondly, research and debate have been largely oriented, at least in the UK, to the issue of managerial control as the perceived focus of labour-capital relations. The consequence of this has been the lack of attention given to the role played by other groups in the configuration of organizational power especially the professions and technical specialists. In sum, labour process theory would appear to be inadequate for the task of analysing professional work within the public sector (Thompson, 1990, pp.110-11). Yet if one is to adequately comprehend the content and consequences of computer-based technologies within hospitals this is precisely what is needed. The next section attempts to resolve this seeming paradox.

Labour process and the public sector The public sector is a critical case for the labour process model because of its historically necessary legitimizing role within all capitalist societies (O'Connor, 1973 1984; Habermas, 1976; Gough, 1979). This role has been challenged in the 1980s and 1990s with privatization and marketization within the public sector giving rise to new discourses of a post-Fordist and post-modern kind (e.g. Flynn, 1992, pp.188-92; Burrows and Loader, 1994; Walby et al., 1994; Dent, 1995b) as well ones relating to the possibility of a new communitarianism to replace both the market and public sector provision (Giddens, 1994; Rustin, 1995). These new debates, whilst reflecting a reconfiguration of the relationship between the state and society, are still concerned with the issue of legitimation. Any labour process analysis of the NHS has to recognise that the service's organizational priorities have been primarily premised on the production of use values, 'however distorted' more than exchange values (Thompson, 1990, p.110). The organization is, consequently, defined primarily by political rather than economic criterion if only because governments rather than markets ultimately make the decisions on resourcing issues. Nevertheless, to exclude, a priori, any state sector organization because it presents complications for labour process theory would seriously weaken the model and limit its applicability to what Thompson (1990, p.108) has referred to as a 'plant particularism' incapable of moving outside the factory gates or the office blocks, leisure complexes and hospitals operating within the private sector.

The professions It is also within the public sector environment that we find the professions have developed a particularly distinct role. Without the market to directly dictate priorities it has been the professions, to a greater or lesser extent, who have been responsible for defining them. To some extent, the relationship between state and the professions would appear to parallel that of *responsible autonomy* as the following quote from Friedman (1977, p.78) indicates:

> [This] type of strategy attempts to harness the adaptability of labour power by giving workers leeway and encouraging them to adapt to changing situations in a manner beneficial to the firm. To do this top managers give workers status, authority and responsibility. [They] try to win their loyalty, and co-opt their organizations to the firm's ideal ... ideologically.

Clearly there are a number of parallels between *responsible autonomy* and professional autonomy not least because the occupational groups thus organized are differentiated from others because of their central role within the division of labour. There is, nevertheless, a crucial difference between the two types of autonomies: *responsible autonomy* is the outcome of management strategies within a context of prevailing labour market conditions and worker resistance (Friedman, 1977) and professional autonomy is the outcome of strategies adopted by the organized occupational groups themselves. These occurred in the nineteenth century before the rise of corporate business and the emergence of the welfare state which was the case with the medical profession (Johnson, 1972, p.52; Larson, 1977). Nurses, by contrast, relied more on a 'collective mobility project' to gain a state recognized professional status in the early part of the twentieth century but theirs was a more circumscribed kind than that of the doctors (Witz, 1992). Computer specialists claim to autonomy post-dates both doctors and nurses and result far more from competition between the computer occupations and managerial groups and did not directly involve the state (Armstrong, 1984, pp.115-16; Murray and Knights, 1990, pp.177-8).

The process of professionalization is significantly affected by strategies adopted by the state. Certain professions can be said to have been explicitly promoted by the capitalist state to meet its requirements of social reproduction. Examples here would include accountants (Johnson, 1972; 1982) and engineers (Larson, 1977). Doctors, by contrast, have been able to define the collaboration between themselves and the state much more than most professions. This has much to do with the dependency of the state on the doctors central role in health care delivery. This contrasts with the other two professional groups considered in this book: nurses and computer specialists. The professionalization of nursing was constrained in a way that doctors never were by direct controls of the state and the cross-cutting reality of patriarchy and gender (Turner, 1987, pp.146-54; Witz, 1993, pp.166-7 and 202-3). Witz (1993, p. 166) goes as far as to argue that the nurses' professionalization project failed but it would be more accurate to say that the nursing profession has been 'shaped' by the professionalizing strategies of doctors - and continues to be so (Davies, 1992, p. 248).

Unlike both doctors and nurses, members of the profession of computer specialists are widely employed in the private as well as the public sectors of the economy. They do not enjoy any occupational monopoly and professional registration is not mandatory. Nevertheless, there is in the UK the British Computer Society (BCS) that takes responsibility for accrediting university and college courses that lead to professional status.

Generally, *responsible autonomy* has been the preferred strategy of the British state towards the professions in the state sector. This, however, would not be an accurate way of describing the actual relationship. In the case of the medical profession doctors have long persisted in pursuing strategies and tactics to prevent their corporate selves being fully incorporated into the state apparatus of health care. This contrasts, as Witz

(1992) has shown, with the professions of nursing and midwifery who remain caught up in an interplay of strategies which circumscribe the their professional autonomies even today. For example, in connection with current ideas of 'new nursing' and nurse training, instead of there being a growth in numbers of autonomous nurse practitioners there pressures have been for nurses to extend their roles in order they can take on tasks previously carried out by junior doctors before their reduction in hours (Walby et al., 1994, pp.77-81).

A central plank of the doctors' strategy has been their claim to clinical autonomy which has enabled them to dominate the organization of nursing and the labour process of health care delivery generally. In sociological terms, clinical autonomy is, essentially, the indetermination component of an indetermination/ technicity (I/T) ratio. It is defined by its lack of definition by the profession (Jamous and Peloille, 1970, p.112). The distinction between a state defined *responsible autonomy* and an independent (i.e. autonomous) status might be said to be that between organizational and institutional control. To explain, organizational control refers to the rules imposed by the state bureaucracy with the intent of limiting the profession's autonomy within their work situation for as Abercrombie and Urry (1983, p.121) have explained, '[b]ureaucracy is ... Janus-faced, for it is a system of constraint, Service class workers benefit from bureaucratic employment in that they have relative autonomy, but they are also relatively constrained by bureaucratic rules'. Professionalization, by contrast, is characterised by an alternative, institutional, mode of control. This refers to the ability of an organized profession to define the extent of its members' autonomy within the work situation. It is important to note, however, that the distinction between organizational and institutional control is, in reality, far from clear-cut. Both types of control are tendencies rather than absolutes. The professional autonomy of doctors is something that has been constantly negotiated and re-negotiated between state and profession since the former has become directly involved in the delivery of health care. Initially, the predominant mode of professional autonomy resulted from the kind of state formations that emerged during the nineteenth century (Johnson, 1982, p.189) when the modern form of the medical profession was established and, subsequently, with the establishment of the Welfare State and the NHS.

The state and the medical profession have been, more or less, continually in conflict over the issue of the cost implications of clinical autonomy since, at least, the mid 1960s with the introduction of the 'Cogwheel' reforms. Negotiations, however, have always taken place within the framework of a centralized health service. Only by restructuring the health service with the introduction of the 'internal market' and thereby separating the allocative and operational decisions (Pahl and Winkler, 1974, pp.114-15) has the administration been able to organizationally undermine the doctors' traditional dominance. As a consequence of these new arrangements doctors are no longer able to commit additional resources as an outcome of their clinical decisions alone (e.g. Klein, 1989, p.83; Flynn, 1992, pp.79-103).

Doctors will retain their control over the work situation (operational decisions), but allocative decisions will now become a managerial prerogative although some doctors in with their new clinical director responsibilities will participate in these decisions. Moreover, it is possible that a cadre of medical managers may eventually become the principal actors in the management decision-making processes. Comparative evidence from Sweden (Coombs and Jonsson, 1991, pp.89-107) and North America (Derber et al., 1990, pp.161-4) would suggest, however, that doctors as managers (e.g. clinical directors) will be most concerned with the financial and management issues directly related to clinical work and its organization rather than the broader concerns of senior management and trust boards. The dividing line between doctoring and managing is no longer a clear cut one and it is perfectly possible that some members of the medical profession will pursue a career as senior medical managers competing with others to try to ensure the continued medical dominance within the health system.

These fundamental changes in the NHS and profession/state relations do not constitute any 'proletarianization' of doctors for as McKinlay and Arches (1985, p.161) have explained they still retain their 'control over certain prerogatives relating to the location, content and essentiality of [their] task activities' (quoted in Elston, 1991, p.63) even if they perceive themselves as suffering a loss of occupational status as Larson (1980) and Derber (1982; Derber et al., 1990, pp.122-5) have argued. Instead doctors are increasingly coming under the organizational control of the state (mediated by the internal market) at the expense of the collective institutional control of the organized profession: a change to what I have called *responsible autonomy.* This modification, however, has not been at the expense of the doctors dominant (patriarchal) position within hospitals, nevertheless, they have had to accept that they are no longer the only arbiters of health care delivery. The establishment of resource management and 'purchaser-provider' relations within the NHS now means that management too has the power to decide which hospitals patients are to be referred. All this adds up to a radical re-adjustment rather than a class revolution.

Technology, social choice and strategies While earlier labour process theorists were concerned to elaborate on Braverman's model within a fully articulated Marxist political economy by the early 1980s a more voluntarist model was emerging. This has been referred to as a social or strategic choice model (Wilkinson, 1983; 17-25; Buchanan, 1983, 1986; Buchanan and Boddy, 1983). Whereas, the earlier variants imported labour market considerations into the analysis the 'social choice' variant is associated with the analysis of technology. It has parallels with the social construction (or 'shaping') of technology as presented by Noble (1979, 1985) although it might more accurately be viewed as the organizational construction of technology. In Noble's case of numerically controlled machines (1977, p.30) the centrality of 'choice' in the analysis stems with his identification of the engineer as the real core to the capitalist labour process rather than the ideology of Scientific Management (Smith, 1987, pp.41-2). This directly links with his concern, to 'show that technology is not an autonomous force impinging upon human affairs from "outside", but is the product of a social process, a historically specific activity carried on by some people, and not others, for particular purposes' (Noble, 1979, p.18). It is in this way that the deskilling potential of new technologies has not, on the whole, taken place. This has been either because the skill grades have been 'hotly contested' by labour unions or, more generally, the degree and reliability of the automation have been insufficient for management to be able to rely wholly on unskilled people (Noble, 1979, pp.41-2; 1985, pp.120-21). Wilkinson's (1983, pp.17-25) UK study draws on Noble's work and shares his general conclusions but in combination with Child's social action concept of strategic choice.

The social choice variant of the labour process effectively deals with the problems associated with technological determinism by stressing the specific social and organizational conditions relating to the design, implementation and utilization of new technologies. It has achieved this, however, only at the expense of losing some generalizability. This can be reclaimed by pressing into service the concept of strategy. The term is, broadly speaking, used within social science discourse as a way of explaining the inter-relations between structure and process which has its roots in game theory (Crow, 1989, pp.1-2). Managerial strategies, or better, organizational strategies (as these would include more than those of management) are a consequence of the contestation of interests relating directly to the management and control of the labour process. This is 'best understood as a political process in which management is no more unified and omniscient than workers are inert and impotent' (Knights and Willmott, 1990, p.13). Strategy has impinged on labour process analysis, at least indirectly, by way of two main influences, firstly, in the form of game theory (Lash and Urry, 1984; Dent, 1991) and, secondly, in the form of Foucault's theory of 'disciplinary power' (1977; Sakolsky, 1992). My argument will be that game theory is ultimately too abstract whereas a Foucauldian approach, despite complications, is not. In order to explain it is to these two theories I now turn.

(a) Game theory

Burawoy's analysis (1979) of workers 'making out' is the most obvious labour process candidate for game theory yet his analysis has little in common with the rationalist game theory I am referring to here. His analysis remains rooted in a fairly structured Bravermanesque version despite his insights into workers active consent in the production process (Knights, 1990, pp.310-11). It is Lash and Urry (1984) who have explored the game theoretic as a means of analysing strategies as benefit-maximising forms of action drawing on the works of Elster (e.g. 1982) and Offe and Wiesenthal (1980). In general terms the game theory model assumes that players have some, but incomplete, knowledge of the other players' resources and intentions. The common example is that of the 'Prisoners' Dilemma' in which two prisoners are, separately, confronted with the 'choice' of likely prison sentences depending on whether they each confess, blame the other, or say nothing (Elster, 1989, pp.28-9; Walters, 1994, p.79). While the players are assumed to make rational choices the consequences of their decisions may be unintended. The model was originally proposed by Olson to explain the logic of collective action (1965) which Elster, in particular, has developed. It is premised on 'an uncompromising methodological individualism' (Hindness, 1988, p.23): individuals are assumed to have the capacity for rational choice but the aggregated outcomes give rise to unintended consequences (Lash and Urry, 1984, p.37; Hindness, 1988, 244). The revised version of the theory propounded by Offe and Wiesenthal explicitly avoids the methodological individualism by making the assumption that organizations do exhibit a collective and purposive identity and are not merely the unintended consequences of aggregated individual decisions (Lash and Urry, 1984, p.40). Whether players are groups, classes or societies they are conceptually irreducible to individuals within the same 'game' for once constituted a game analysis involves the reification of the collectivities involved. A consequence of this is that the analyzes are only tenuously and abstractly related to actual conduct (Giddens, 1984, p.313). Despite, or because, of this limitation the general model has a usefulness in its ability to simplify complexity and clarify the issues. Clearly the game-theoretic can only ever be, at best, a partial model for it oversimplifies the relations between the game players. Elias, avoids this problem by arguing that 'these [games] models of interweaving are not theoretical in the customary sense of the word. They are didactic models ...' (1978, pp.91-2); the model is used as an aid to explanation and not an explanation in itself. For such an explanation it is useful to turn to the work of Foucault.

(b) Strategy and disciplinary power

More recently a post-structuralist tendency can be discerned within at least some labour process discourse. Much of it has developed as a response to the widespread implementation of Just In Time (JIT) and Total Quality Management (TQM) which are perceived to parallel the rationale of the nineteenth century panopticon (e.g. Sewell and Wilkinson, 1992, pp.271-89). The appropriateness of a Foucauldian analysis here is reasonably obvious. *Discipline and Punish* (Foucault, 1977) offers an analytical framework of *responsible autonomy* as a management control (discipline) strategy. Unlike labour process analysis, however, there is no privileging of production or paid labour. Power relations are not manifested as a struggle between the exploiters and exploited but as a web of complex relations that have given rise to 'a plurality of disciplinary mechanisms, techniques of surveillance and power-knowledge strategies' (Knights, 1990, p.319). This post-structuralist extension of labour process analysis has been particularly associated with the work of Knights (1990; Knights and Vurdubakis, 1994) who has argued:

> Foucault's analysis is not a substitute for theories of domination and exploitation [i.e. labour process theory] it ... presents a conception of power and subjectivity that facilitates an understanding of how subjects voluntarily engage in practices which reproduce patriarchal and capitalist institutions (1990, p.327).

Whether this importation of post-structuralist agnosticism is strictly compatible with the emancipatory intent of labour process theory is itself a contestable issue (Thompson, 1993). Foucault has said, 'I am neither an adversary nor a partisan of Marxism' (Rabinow, 1984, p.355) but, as Knights (1990, p.323) has pointed out, 'Foucault has been at great pains .... to purge discourse of the pre-given, universal subject as the foundation of truth and meaning and as the starting point of analysis'. Nevertheless, while there is a strong rejection of any humanistic essentialism or emancipation as an enlightenment project within Foucault's work there is a strong sense that human action is inherently free even if always entrapped within a complex net of power inter-relations. This begins to read like a recast version of game theory but this time without any *a priori* notion of rationality (e.g. Knights, 1990, p.326).

The intention has been to recast labour process analysis so that it can break free of the determinism of its origins but retains its particular focus on work processes as the site of control, exploitation and accumulation. There is one more perspective to be considered known generically as social constructionism. Here it is the artefact rather more than the artizan that is privileged in the analysis.

The social construction of technology

The social construction of technology is an all inclusive term that incorporates a wide range of approaches which share the assumption that technology is to varying degrees socially 'shaped'. Some variants of labour process theory can be included (e.g. Noble, 1985) as well as several feminist writers on technology (e.g. Cockburn, 1985; Barker and Downing, 1985; Wajcman, 1991) and all the other writers also included in the MacKenzie and Wacjman's seminal collection 'The Social Shaping of Technology' (1985). The term has been adopted by work of Pinch and Bijker (1987) whereas other sociological writers also interested in this subject matter have preferred to avoid using this term. I am particularly thinking here of Callon (1986) and Latour (1987) prefer to use the term 'actor networks' for reasons that will be made clear later. All, nevertheless, adhere to the premiss that technology is a 'seamless web' (Hughes, 1986) of the social, economic, political and technological (Bijker et al., 1987, pp.10-11). Although, Hughes conceptualises this in systems terms (1987, pp.51-83) in contra-distinction to Callon and Latour's approach which is network based. In Hughes' case (1987, p.53) there is a distinction to be made between system and environment whereas in the case of actor networks 'there is no outside/inside (that is, social/technology) dichotomy' (Bijker et al., 1987, p.12) and this indicates less consensus and more complexity within the 'social constructionist' school than might initially appear to be the case.

Before exploring the internal variations between these theoreticians of technology it is important to point out that they have had a wider impact on sociology than might at first be apparent. Their influence has extended beyond the sociologies of science and technology and is currently impacting on the sociology of organizations and work (Clegg, 1989, pp.202-7; Grint, 1991, pp.148-50; Law, 1991). Bloomfield et al (1990, 1992a), for instance, have utilized the actor network and fabrication of technology concepts to analyze the NHS Resource Management Initiative.

It will be useful to start with the works of Callon (1986, 1987) and Latour (1987). Their general approach is one committed to empirically finding out how specific scientific research and technological development work activities are actually carried out in all their messy complexity. To employ one of their favourite metaphors, the aim is to open up the 'black box' of the research laboratory and technology departments. As Latour explains (1987, p.3):

> The word black box is used by cyberneticians whenever a piece of machinery or set of commands is too complex. In its place they draw a little box about which they need to know nothing but its input and output ... [N]o matter how controversial their history, how complex their inner workings, how large their commercial or academic networks that hold them in place, only their input and output count.

In order to open up 'black boxes' Callon and Latour rely on the metaphor of the heterogenous network (Law, 1992). In their version actors are heterogeneous entities that constitute a network (Bijker et al., 1987, p.11) which also includes non-human entities such as 'machines, animals, texts, money, architectures - any material you can care to mention' (Law, 1992, p.381). This approach is not restricted to technological artefacts but has claims to be a theory of social order which overcomes the basic 'structure', 'agency' problem of sociology (Callon and Latour, 1981; Law, 1986, p.382). A good illustration of the approach is Callon's paradigmatic case of the scallops and fisherman of St Briec Bay (1986, pp.196-233). The scallops and their larvae, as well as the fishermen are 'actors' in the heterogenous network of scallop harvesting. Thus, Latour writes (with or without irony): 'Threatened by starfish and fishermen, ignored for years by oceanographers who do not even know if they are able to move or not, the animal is slowly disappearing from the bay. Whom should the scallops' larvae tie themselves to so as to resist their enemies?' (Latour, 1987, p.203) . The answer according to Latour is a group of Japanese scientists but that is not of central concern here. What is crucial is that the case study of the French scallop is premised on an agnostic Machiavellianism and free association. In other words, the analyst is impartial in the treatment of all actors in a controversy whether they are human or non-human, animate or inanimate (this has intriguing ramification for the notion of actor as subject - what does it feel to be a scallop?).

The general approach is known as the 'sociology of translation' or, more descriptively, 'sociology of enrolment' (Clegg, 1989, p.203). It is categorically an empirical approach that avers any moralist content. This means that interests are seen as the 'temporarily stabilized outcomes of previous processes of enrolment [to a network]' (Callon and Law, 1982, p.622 quoted in Clegg, 1989, p.204). In other words, it is not necessary to ascribe intention. The approach is as much a theory of power as it is about science and technology and the method seeks to identify how actors (and actants) 'translate' intent into resources and resources into networks of control (Clegg, 1989, p.204). There are four 'moments' of this translation:

1. Problematization (or 'how to become indispensable').
2. Intéressement (or 'how allies are locked in place').
3. Enrolment (or 'how to define and co-ordinate the roles').
4. Mobilization of allies.

While these were elaborated in the scallops' case study they can equally well be applied to healthcare computing:

1. *Problematization* involves the advocates of healthcare computing claiming that their policies are indispensable to the future efficiency of health care organization and provision.

2 The *Intéressement* 'moment' is when the advocates are able to sufficiently interest other actors (and actants) in their programme that they are willing to be enrolled within the computerization programme 'network'.

3. *Enrolment* refers to the set of strategies designed to define and interrelate the various roles into alliances and coalitions.

4. *Mobilization* relates to the set of methods used to try and ensure that members of the alliances and coalitions do not betray the general strategy.

Any actor network, however, is unable to reproduce itself because they are - by their very nature - fragile and transient although they can extend their life by being inscribed in material form, e.g. architecture (Latour, 1988, pp.36-7; Grint, 1990, p.150) or computer systems. This constant need to maintain a network ('inscription')or replace a failed one has many parallels with Foucault's conceptualization of power as the 'effect' of social relationships. The model generally is rich in post-structuralist potential even if the authors themselves do not acknowledge this point (Clegg, 1989, pp.16-17). This can be illustrated by reference to *Discipline and Punish* in which Foucault (1977) argues that power is necessarily conceived of as possessing a disciplinary, rather than sovereign and this is further reinforced in the *History of Sexuality* where he proposes' ... power is exercised from innumerable points, in the interplay of nonegalitarian and mobile relations' (1981, p.94). Just as with Callon (1986) and Latour (1987, pp.124-5) Foucault too draws on Machiavelli's writings in his analysis of power-relations:

> In this way we will escape from the system of Law-and-Sovereign which has captivated political thought for such a long time. And if it is true that Machiavelli was among the few ... who conceived the power of the Prince in terms of force relationships, perhaps we need to go one step further, do without the persona of the Prince, and decipher power mechanisms on the basis of a strategy that is immanent in force relations (Foucault, 1981, p.97)

This intellectual parallelism between Foucault, on the one hand, and Latour and Callon, on the other, means that specific studies of science and technology can be incorporated within a broader analysis of social and organizational change. At the same time, however, this very facility gives rise to three specific problems: (a) the conflation of scientific and political discourses (Amsterdamska, 1990, p.502); (b) technological determinism; (c) reification (Berger and Luckman, 1971, pp.106-9). In order to address these issues I will discuss, first, Pinch and Bijker's version of Social Construction of Technology (SCOT), a version that analytically keeps technology and power separate. Second, Bloomfield's (1995) rationale for the inclusion of non-human actants which directly addresses the question of power and determinism and in the process implicitly deals with reification.

(a) Science, technology and power: Pinch and Bijker In contrast to both Callon and Latour, Pinch and Bijker (1984, 1987) have little to say on the issue of power even though it is implicitly present in the discussion on 'closure'. Their approach draws instead on the 'Empirical Programme of Relativism' (EPOR) which asserts that there are three stages in scientific explanation. Firstly, scientific findings exhibit interpretative flexibility (i.e. open to more than one interpretation). Second, this interpretative flexibility is 'resolved' by way of closure mechanisms by which the scientific debate is presented to the public as having been resolved. This third stage, of relating the closure mechanism to the wider social-cultural milieu, has not yet been carried out in study of contemporary science (Pinch and Bijker, 1987, p.27). It is not clear whether this 'oversight' is a methodological problem for EPOR or a characteristic of science (i.e. 'social' - as opposed to 'scientific' - closure is either not a high priority or takes a very long time to establish). The case of technology is slightly different. Pinch and Bijker have adapted EPOR to

the study of technology and called it the social construction of technology (SCOT). The task of those engaged in the SCOT programme is to open the 'black box' of technology in a manner synonymous with EPOR in the natural sciences in order to identify and analyze the social processes of artefacts. In the Pinch and Bijker's now classic case the artefact was the bicycle (1984, 1987). The SCOT method brings together three basic concepts derived from EPOR which are as follows.

(i) interpretative flexibility
(ii) closure mechanisms
(iii) social group

Each of these will now be briefly explained in turn:

(i) *Interpretative flexibility* Technological artefacts are not givens but are culturally constructed. Pinch and Bijkerand, in their case study of the pneumatic tyre demostrate that it was originally introduced as an improvement of a bicycle's suspension but it only became widely adopted once it was realised that it was a means of making the safety bicycle travel faster - its function had been re-interpretted (see *Closure by redefinition* below).

(ii) *Closure mechanisms* Closure mechanisms refer to the 'the stabilization of an artefact' (i.e. its general acceptability) (Pinch and Bijker, 1984, p.424; 1987, p.44). Only two types are described, although there is no reason to preclude others (1984, pp.426-7):

- rhetorical.
- redefinition.

In the case of 'rhetorical closure', technical problems are not resolved in the usual sense of the word. Instead members of the core set (e.g. manufacturers, engineers, advertisers) publicly asserting that the artefact works splendidly. This clearly invites analysis in terms of power and influence but these authors remain focused on meanings and interpretations as if the discourse had no power implications. Thus, for instance, the claim of early computer manufactures that main frame batch processing systems were essential for any forward thinking company overlooked to mention the constraints such systems imposed on organizations in terms of inflexibility. A situation that existed until the introduction of the mini-computer (e.g. Burnett and Nolan, 1975, pp.148-56). 'Closure by redefinition' occurs when an artefact is functionally redefined differently to its original purpose. The example used by Pinch and Bijker is that of the pneumatic tyres for bicycles. These tyres were originally designed as an anti-vibration device for the small wheeled 'safety' bicycles but was only commonly accepted when they were seen, in practice, to enable cyclist to reach high speeds. This in turn spelt the demise of the 'penny farthing' bicycle for not only could their small wheeled competitors now reach higher speeds they were also significantly easier and safer to ride (Pinch and Bijker, 1987, pp.42-3 and 45).

In the case of computing the dominance of the mainframe machines limited the implementation of the 'user-friendly' windows, icons, mouse and pulldown menus (WIMPs) interface for over a decade. The interface was originally developed, along with 'object-oriented programming' by Xerox at their Palo Alto Research Centre during the 1970s but their practical and market value was not recognised until personal computing began to seriously erode the mainframe systems dominance in the business market (Forester, 1987, pp.205-7). In the event it was a relative newcomer to the industry, Apple Computing, that became famous for introducing these more accessible interfaces and flexible programming in their computers (LISA and Macintosh) (Weinberg, 1990, p.31).

(iii) *Social Groups* The term refers to any relevant institution, organization or organized or even unorganized groups of individuals.'The key requirement is that all members of a certain social group share the same set of meanings, attached to a specific artefact.' (Pinch and Bijker, 1987, p.31) . The identification of such groups could be a rather daunting task as there are typically a large number of groups involved especially when one moves outside the R & D laboratories (1984, p.431). Moreover, the relevant social groups may well be heterogeneous in the meanings they attach to the artefact (1987, pp.32-4). In terms of the early development to the bicycle there were a range of issues that, in turn, had their pro- and anti-lobbyists and innovators; penny farthings vs small wheeled bicycles in terms of speed, safety, and comfort (1987, p.37). Bicycles for women were also viewed by many as an important issue (ibid.).

The artefact of the bicycle, however, is fairly straightforward when compared to a whole range of new technologies typically comprising of a complex set of networks of high technology components and social and organizational arrangements which can be extremely difficult delineate. In the case of computer-based information systems, besides the hardware, the peripherals, cabling and communications, there are the programmes and packages (software), the programmers, designers and analysts. In addition to all this there are the policy makers and managers and users and the funders of the systems (Checkland, 1981; Willcocks and Mason, 1987, pp.10-11). Yet despite their limitations the concepts of 'closure by redefinition' and 'rhetorical closure' remain useful means of summarizing the state of many computer systems and programmes.

(b) and (c) Technological systems and outcomes Bloomfield (1995, p.497) argues that technology is not the cause of organizations but its outcome. Thus the actor network perspective does not imply technological determinism nor systems reification. First, so the argument runs, technology 'is the result of the formation of networks of non-human (artefacts) and

human actants'. Thus, to use a hospital example, radiology technology which now includes computer-assisted X-ray tomography (CAT) scanners, nuclear magnetic resonance (NMR), positron emission tomography (PET) to name just three variants (Weinberg, 1990, pp.121-22). None of these determine the organization of radiology or its role within the broader hospital division of labour although the size and cost of some of these artefacts will have a significant influence.

Second, the non-human actants are not to be viewed as reified outcomes of human activity but 'delegated' devices (artefacts) which stand in for humans who might otherwise perform the task. The example he cites is the use of 'sleeping policemen' as traffic calming devices. Here the hump in the road stands in for a human police officer. In the case of an automated hospital information system the computer software stands in for a number of clerks and administrators. These artefacts do not control social relations they 'presuppose, mediate and reinforce them' (op cit., p.497). Moreover, they do so in line with the script provided by humans (ibid., p.498). This leads Bloomfield to assert that delegation is always 'context dependent' which is an important sociological caveat.

Third, it is not possible in advance to determine the outcomes of actor networks as the dynamic complexity of any new arrangement gives rise to new issues, problems and relations not previous considered. This is also true of hospital information systems (see Chapter 3) but even in the much simpler case of 'sleeping policemen' unintended consequences have occurred. Whilst, traffic has been calmed new problems have been identified including increased exhaust fumes and their unsuitability for ambulances carrying very sick patients. Such innovations are always contestable.

Finally, Bloomfield argues that we should be careful in taking on board the case of durability. Here he is trying to avoid an excessive reliance on power as the determinant of technology outcomes for as Amsterdamska (1987, p.502) has sharply pointed it can lead to one being 'indifferent to the means and methods of enrolment and control' (Amsterdamska, 1987, p.502) with the logical consequence that an actor network analysis would identify the Lysenko dialectical biology as the work of a great scientist! Bloomfield not so much revises the concepts of durability and delegation as modifies the emphases as between power and technology. Durability, he argues, is not given forever, nor is it constantly threatened by any dramatic instability. To illustrate the point he offers the example of digital telecommunications. Whilst these are more durable than analogue ones if they fail they do so catastrophically. Analogue systems by contrast are fairly robust and can continue to deliver some kind of signal even though very distorted. The implications for those within organizations who are increasingly delegating their information systems to the safe-keeping of digital computer systems have not escaped the imagination of science fiction writers - including the script writers of the popular Canadian series 'X-Files'. In their first series there was an episode in which a computer system adopted the characteristics of HAL in the film '2001: Space Odyssey' and attempted to entrap and kill all humans who threatened its viability. This example, however, lies in the world of fantasy. Life support and monitoring systems using micro-chip technologies within intensive therapy units (ITU) are examples, on the other hand, that do not. They are real and malfunctions within these systems can have tragic consequences for those whose lives literally depend upon the technology. The point here is that the delegation (and inscription) of technological systems is not a once and for all act. These durable technological systems only continue to function reliability if part of actor networks that uses and relies on them.

Social construction of technological systems: recapitulation

The actor networks of Callon and Latour and the social construction of technology approach of Pinch and Bijker's can be viewed as sub-sets of a common discourse on the social construction of technological systems even if Latour, (1993, pp.51-4) in particular, would find such an appellation perverse. The SCOT approach in separating the artefact and the actors as well as the organization(s) and the(ir) environment(s) makes for a more structured and less complex model than actor network theory. Moreover, whilst Pinch and Bijker's model lacks the theoretical sophistication of their Gallic colleagues it is, nevertheless, able to specify the means by which technological artefacts - including hospital computers - are designed, introduced and utilized without reducing the account to socially determinist explanation. Latour, as one of the main protagonists for actor network theory, argues for a more realist position and is critical of the social determinism of the social constructionists' analysis of technology. It is in order to avoid this social determinism that partly accounts for why Latour includes actants into the actor network and the fabrication of technology.

Actor networks are based on an ongoing and all-inclusive process of 'translation' which occurs only if or when the artefact is sufficiently 'taken for granted'. This device conflates technology, non-human life forms and social actors within the same network of power relations except where there is a clear distinction made between the human actor and the delegated non-human actant as Bloomfield suggests. This Latour fails to do preferring instead to see '[h]uman nature [as] the set of its delegates and its representatives, its figures and its messengers'. (Latour, 1993, p.138) and all part of a symmetrical universe of nature and society. Moreover, by including within the explanation that which is to be explained the approach is tautological (Amsterdamska, 1990, p. 497). Pinch and Bijker's model might appear to offer a way around these problems with its focus on the artefact by (a) retaining a divide between artefact and social environment and (b) suggesting a typification schema for closure and stabilization mechanisms (i.e. 'rhetorical' and 'redefinition'). By this device the technology is real but the nature and degree of its acceptance and use (closure) that is socially defined. This avoids the problems of tautology and conflation but presents the researcher with another problem, identified earlier, of delineating a complex and extended set of networks. One way of avoiding these difficulties would be to stay with actor network theory but adopt the revisions suggested by Bloomfield (1995) and prioritizing the human actor over the artefact or technological system for despite these criticisms and reservations actor network theory provides a powerful framework within which to develop an analysis of information and communications technologies.

Conclusions

The chapter started with a selective and critical review of the health care computing literature identifying the main strands and how these related to sociological research into organizations and computing. This led me to a consideration of labour process theory as a paradigm for understanding hospital organization and health care computing. I argued that with some modifications the model did provide a means of analysing healthcare computing systems and professional work. But the approach, because of its underlying assumptions, treats computing technology as a 'black box'. It is for this reason that the latter third of the chapter was devoted to the social construction or 'shaping' of technology literature. Here the works of Callon and Latour, Pinch and Bijker were discussed. A Foucauldian post-structuralism was identified as providing a common thread in the analysis of power relations within the actor network paradigm and some tendencies within labour process discourse.

The rest of this book is concerned with understanding the dynamics and relations as between computer systems, NHS hospitals' organization and control. The chapters dealing with these different elements will draw variously from the discussion presented here.

Notes

1. The research literature on innovation is much broader than being referred to here in relation to healthcare computing. For a more comprehensive discussion see, for example, Clark and Staunton (1989).

2. The term 'social construction of technological systems' is used here generically and is not restricted to the specific Social Construction of Technology (SCOT) approach associated with Pinch and Bijker (1984, 1987).

3 Computers, management strategies and the state

Introduction

It is the issue of the diffusion of healthcare computing - which was introduced in the previous chapter - that is to be discussed here. This time the focus is upon the role played by management strategies in the process. The NHS hospital sector in the 1960s played a central role in the then government's policy of using public sector organizations to support and stimulate the market for the main UK computer company - ICL. A company formed from the merging of ICT and English Electric in 1968. Under this policy certain hospitals were to pioneer new systems which once proven would be introduced into all hospitals. Rationally this approach made sense. It shares some of the assumptions of the 'bandwagon' model outlined by McLoughlin and Clark (1994, p. 13) in which new technology once successfully pioneered is taken up by 'mature' firms and industries not able to develop the innovations themselves. What was once new and unusual becomes the norm for the industry. In the NHS, however, the healthcare computing 'bandwagon' never really gained momentum. Not, at least, in terms of the technology and systems although the healthcare computing literature 'bandwagon' did and has provided a rich source of information for this chapter. This early period which starts with the introduction of the first mainframes, batch processing, systems of the late 1950s is, however, only one component of the chapter. Centre stage is reserved for the analysis of the computer and information systems strategies within the NHS which are discussed in light of the 'stages of growth models' that information specialists draw upon to make sense of the policies and processes. The case study is based on the events within one health region although material is drawn from other health regions and elsewhere too. The advantage of not painting on too broad a canvas is that the 'stages' will be easier to identify without the need of extensive qualifications for the different circumstances of each region health authority (RHA). My basic argument will be that computerization in hospitals has developed as the outcome of the interplay of interests of the British computer industry, central government and computer interests internal to the NHS. It was not developed initially as part of any managerial strategy to improve the efficiency or effectiveness of the NHS although such outcomes where hoped for. Before taking the argument any further, however, it will be useful to make some distinctions between the different types of computer systems used within hospitals.

Types of hospital computing

Hospital computing is currently organized or being developed to support the following information systems (e.g. Bloomfield and Coombs, 1992, p.470):

1. *Patient administration systems* used to record and monitor the admission, movements and discharge of patients. The name of the consultant in charge will also be included and possibly diagnosis.

2. *Departmental systems* are the systems used by specialist departments, such as X-Ray and pathology but including nursing. These are systems designed to schedule work and record results.

3. *Order communications systems* refer to ward systems that interface with the departmental systems. These provide direct communications of orders and test results between the two.

4. *Medical audit systems* are designed to capture and then analyse clinical data for the regular auditing of clinical practice.

5. *Case mix systems (resource management systems)* are designed to generate information on patterns of resource usage associated with the treatment of patients in different specialities and under different consultants

At present, the main emphasis is on implementation of integrated hospital-wide systems that will primarily provide detailed information on costs and resource usage for each type of patient in the process. This policy follows from and builds on introduction resource management within the NHS. Currently there are two main approaches to any computer strategy designed to underpin this new integrated network strategy: the *Big Bang* or *incrementalism.* Before discussing this recent policy debate it is informative to look at the history of hospital computing over the last thirty years. This is interesting in policy terms as many of the arguments now being made been used before. Sociologically this is also interesting for it permits a longitudinal study of professionals use or otherwise of computing. If the original work on the 1960s computer-based systems was intended to create automated medical records as the cornerstone of a hospital-wide system why is it we still do not have any such systems in wide-scale use? For instance, Michael Cross in the *Health Services Journal* (26 January 1995, p.1) argues that the NHS Executive must work harder to promote electronic patient records and on the face of it so they should. But the same point was being made by John Anderson back in the 1960s (The Times, 5 October 1982, p.13) the NHS failed then why should it not do so again? The big difference between the earlier period and the present one which may make electronic patient records a reality is not technological but the introduction of the internal (or quasi-) market. Today NHS hospital systems have to include data on the cost and resource implications of patient care this was not originally the case. Earlier computing was driven by wider considerations and it is useful to refer to a simple taxonomy in order to explain. This can be provided by Holoien (1977) who, in writing on hospital computing in the USA makes the unsurprising distinction between administrative and clinical systems. The first refers to matters as payroll, patient admissions, supplies and any other matters that lie in the province of the administration. Within the NHS, and with the exception of admissions, these responsibilities were not those of the hospitals but of the regional and district authorities. The NHS hospital, at that time, was the operational end of a highly centralized and formal organizational structure. Patients' admissions were recorded on a patient administration system (PAS) (if there was one) which was to form the 'backbone' of the earlier approach to hospital computerization. The second, the clinical systems, refers to medical and nursing systems as well as technical and scientific services. Under this heading are included the medical records which are ambiguously 'clinical' in content but defined as 'administrative' in terms of their legal status (Home Office, 1978, p.69). These records are of particular interest here because they constitute the medical information system and thereby play a crucial role in the organization and delivery of medical care. Moreover, many proponents of hospital computing imagined that the new computer-based patient administration systems would be extended to become automated medical record systems. This did not happen for reasons to be explained later.

Despite being a useful gambit for opening up the discussion, Holoien's systems dichotomy (administrative/clinical) is a limited one. Firstly, it fails to identify adequately the occupational groups or services which are the major users of the various systems. Medical information systems primarily support the work of doctors and may well be linked in to a medical record system. Nursing systems, on the other hand, are not usually linked in with the medical records. Finally, the technical and scientific staff will typically have access to entirely separate computer systems. These systems might be integrated within one hospital information system but functionally they have always been separate. In other words, one can categorize hospital computer systems into four groups according to who will predominantly use them:

1. Administrative systems
2. Technical and scientific support systems

3. Medical information systems
4. Nursing systems.

While three of these categories (2-4) are clinical (and therefore fit Holoien's basic distinction) it is more useful to subdivide according to who are the major occupational users of the system. The reason for this relates to the question of occupational control and medical dominance (Freidson, 1970), concepts deriving from the sociology of professions and which are particularly relevant to our understanding of the design and usage of hospital computer systems. These issues were, at least partly, recognised in the deliberations of the Joint Working Party on the Organization of Medical Work in Hospital who categorized information systems as being either (a) controlled or (b) used but not controlled by doctors (Goldsmith and Mason, 1974, p.174).

My argument here is that doctors have had a significant influence on the development of hospital computing its inception but it was not the result of any organized strategy by the profession. The actor network was more extensive including government ministers and civil servants, a certain computer manufacturing company and their computers and early software. The network also includes the NHS computer specialists and management services personnel chiefly responsible for the implementation and evaluation of these systems.

The analysis I will present here will be of the emergence and growth of IT within the NHS and will be based on a particular periodization. There are on the face of it some parallels here with the 'stages of growth' models that have proven particularly influential within information systems discourse (see Galliers and Sutherland, 1991). In order to clarify the argument I will first consider the 'stages of growth' model and their inappropriateness before turning the history of hospital computing.

'Stages of growth' models and managerial strategies

In a key article by Galliers and Sutherland (1991, pp.92-6) Nolan's classic four and six staged models (as well as three others not discussed here) are reviewed. The four stages of the original model (Gibson and Nolan, 1974) were as follows:

1. Initiation (typically within accounts department)
2. Contagion (development of applications for other functions)
3. Control (budgetary and quality controls set in place by senior management)
4. Maturity.

In general terms what the stages express is a period of early, largely unplanned growth under loose budgetary controls with computer managers having considerable autonomy. By Stage 3, however, computer budgets were seen by senior management to be 'out of control' (i.e. excessive) and there was a strong move to centralize the computing function (referred to in the earlier articles as EDP or Electronic Data Processing) under strong budgetary, technical and organizational controls. (Gibson and Nolan, 1974, p.79). These three stages reflected the historical development of computing from the late 1950s until the early 1970s in the US The fourth stage was more speculative-cum-utopian it being defined as a resource-oriented planning and control system. Within this system the computer (EDP) manager is elevated board level while systems analysts and programmers are moved out of centralized computer departments and into the user areas. This latter move designed to make the specialists more responsive to the users. Overall, the strategy would have the effect of enhancing the control of senior management (by incorporating the computer manager) whilst fragmenting the occupational control of the computer specialists.

The problems with managing the computing (EDP) function was not so easily resolvable and, according to Nolan (1979) reached 'crisis' proportions by the end of the 1970a. Nolan recommended interposing the following two additional stages between the Control and Maturity stages of his earlier model:

4. Integration
5. Data administration

In part this represented a recognition that the utopia of 'maturity' was not to be easily won. It also represented an awareness that to control computing it is not the technology that management would need to focus but the information and data. As Galliers and Sutherland (1991, pp.90-1) point out 'in addition [to the technology], there are four major growth processes that can be analyzed to identify the organization's stage of maturity' (p.90):

1. extending the scope of the applications portfolio[1] throughout the organization;

2. refocusing the organization of the computer function from being a centralized, 'closed shop' to data resource management;

3. a change in planning and control from an internal focus in the first three stages to an external focus in the latter stages;

4. an increase in the level of user awareness to a point where it has become the driving force for change.

The main point Galliers and Sutherland are making is that Nolan's approach is too influenced by a concern for the interests of senior management rather than the problems confronting the computing managers and professionals.

They are critical of Nolan for overlooking the 'beleaguered DP manager attempting to create a successful I[nformation] S[ystems] function within the organization' (ibid., p.90) for this, as much as any other reason, Galliers and Sutherland provide their own alternative 'stages of growth' model which also has six stages:

1. 'Adhocracy'
2. Starting the foundations
3. Centralized dictatorship
4. Democratic dialectic and co-operation
5. Entrepreneurial opportunity
6. Integrated harmonious relationships

Stage 1: 'Adhocracy' is the initial and relatively uncontrolled stage in which simple applications are introduced (usually accounting systems). Any systems development tends to be ad hoc. Most technical help can be provided by the computer manufacturer's own technical support and 'help line' where computer staff are employed they consist of one or a small number of programmers. There is no real organizational structure associated with IT at this stage.

Stage 2: Starting the foundations marks the beginning of the ascendancy of an IT 'priesthood' in the organization (ibid., p.101). The organization now begins to develop applications for areas other than finance and accounting. A separate IT section comes into existence with a manager appears who is usually responsible to the financial controller or equivalent. Analysts and designers begin to join the IT staff who tend to view user friendliness as 'idiot proofing' and resent user involvement since they appear to constantly change their minds (ibid., p.102).

Stage 3: Centralized dictatorship marks the stage where attempts are made to co-ordinate and centrally control IT within the organization. There is now a computer/IT department which attempts to exercise tight 'top down' control on systems development. Staffing grows and now includes information systems planners and data-base and data administration staff. The manager's title may change to Information Systems Manager or similar. Nevertheless, the department continues to remain out of touch with users leading to problems with systems implementation and acceptance (ibid., p.104) .

Stage 4: Democratic dialectic and co-operation The computer/IT department becomes a little less centralized in a bid to become more responsive to users (and improve the acceptability and usability of systems). The manager is increasingly subordinated to a new Information Systems manager who has business management experience and may not come from an IT background (ibid., p.105). The IT function now becomes federalized with user departments gaining control over systems. Typically, small scale

IT departments are spread throughout the organizations in order to better service the user departments. Meanwhile, it is the Information Services/Management Department that co-ordinates the use of IT throughout the organization. There is now greater integration and co-ordination between systems across the organization. IT staff are joined by the early version of the 'hybrid' the business analyst (See Chapter 4). More generally, the technical skills of IT staff, while still required, are de-emphasized in relation to business skills (ibid., p.106).

Stage 5: Entrepreneurial opportunity Having established the major operational systems the IT players seek opportunities for strategic use of IT. Centralized computer/IT departments have now fully disappeared and computing and information systems resources are spread throughout the organization in various coalitions with the business units. IT is now more market oriented than ever before and decision support systems (DSS) or management information systems (MIS) for senior management are developed and implemented. Under this regime the new role is for the Information Systems planner (ibid., p.108) responsible for the strategic planning of information systems. These specialists come from a 'hybrid' background (see Chapter 4) and are cross-disciplinary in their approach.

Stage 6: Integrated harmonious relationships IT is now deeply embedded throughout every aspect of the organization. It has become 'IT dependent' (Earl, 1989, p.6). Senior management's strategy is the maintenance of comparative strategic advantage and this involves constantly re-assessing all uses of IT. Head of IT now becomes a full member of the board of directors to ensure IT is fully incorporated within the strategic thinking of the organization. Systems development turns more to *inter*-organizational systems (suppliers, customers, government, etc.) to further improve strategic advantage and efficiency. The federal structure of IT function now comes under central scrutiny and co-ordination but in the general 'tight-loose' sense of Peters and Waterman (1982) not in terms of any 'top down' dictatorship.The emphasis is on inter-dependence rather than specialist exclusivity.

These 'stages of growth' models are ubiquitous in information systems literature. They do appear to be useful in identifying the rational and orderly way the development of computer-based information systems. Moreover, the Nolan and the Galliers and Sutherland versions do provide a summary and some insight into the 'state of play' in computing/ IT organization at the time of production (i.e. Nolan = mid 1970s, Galliers and Sutherland = 1990s). There are, however, problems with the general model despite Galliers and Sutherland (1991) attempt to update and amend it. First, there is the confusion over the model's explanatory status. Second, is the problem of time and sequence. Third, the model is inherently utopian.

Concerning the explanatory status of the model, this is one it shares with much of systems theory. Just as is the case with systems models the 'stages of growth' model is a heuristic device which too often comes to be seen, erroneously, as the reality the methodology is intended to reveal. The evolution of IT is a more open and contingent process than Nolan or Galliers and Sutherland suggest. Relatedly, neither model adequately periodizes the stages and this leads me to my second point. The assumption within these models is that stages of growth are followed sequentially. Thus, the earlier experience of those organizations deemed to be approaching maturity (or 'integrated harmonious relationships') constitute the initial stages for other organizations as well. But, an organization at an early stage of IT development may not wish to follow the path set by the more established players. Changes in the economy, technology, organizational design or in society at large could well change the whole logic of the staged progression. Finally, the assumption that there is a stage of 'maturity' (Nolan) or 'integrated harmonious relationships' (Galliers and Sutherland) is utopian and ignores the open-ended and multi-layered reality of organizations in much the same way as systems theory (see Chapter 2, pp.13-14). In light of these problems it would be better not to elevate the epochs in systems development into a prescriptive universal 'stages of growth' schema. Instead it is more useful to identify different periods according to their own internal coherence which may have much in common with other organizations but not for any essentialist reasons. The following periodization of hospital computing is based on this line of reasoning.

The story of hospital computing with the NHS

Computer systems were first introduced into the NHS in the 1950s. In terms of computer and IT strategies the subsequent history can be periodized into four principle stages:

1. Ad hoc (up until 1966)
2. NHS Experimental Computer Programme (1967-81)
3. Corporate systems vs information management (1981-)
4. Networks (circa 1986-).

These stages have broadly paralleled the following management structures and policies within the district health authorities.

1. Hospital management
2. Consensus management
3. General management
4. Resource management.

During the first two stages the inter-connections between computer strategies and management structures at the level of the district health authority or the hospital could best be described as accidental. It largely depended, so I have been told by those working in the area at the time, upon whether or not there were individuals interested enough in hospital computing to develop projects and lobby for resources. Subsequently the district health authorities (DHAs) and hospital management were to become more directly involved in the shaping of the overall strategy. With the shift in emphasis ICL became increasingly challenged by other computer vendors as were the 'in-house' computer specialists who underwent radical changes in their employment arrangements. The reasons for these changes and the processes by which they came about will now be examined in more detail in terms of the four stage periodization:

Stage 1: Ad hoc computing The first data-processing facilities had been introduced into the accounts departments in the mid and late 1950s when punch card systems were introduced (Lamb, 1973, p.37; Barber and Abbott, 1972, p.3). This paralleled the path of computing in commercial and industrial organizations (e.g. Mumford and Banks, 1967, p.175; Gibson and Nolan, 1974, p.77; Nolan, 1979, pp.115-26). In relation to clinical computing it was not really until the 1960s when doctors began to show some interest in developing computer-based clinic record systems (Anderson, 1984, pp.108-11). Few of them were familiar with the technology and had to rely almost wholly on the computer specialists for the development of any systems (ibid., p.109). Two of the best known of these developments of hospital computing during the 1960s were the systems at Kings College (Opit and Woodroffe, 1970; The Times, 5 October 1982, p.13) and The London Hospital (Barber and Abbott, 1972). Some of these systems almost certainly had nursing involvement but specific nursing applications were not developed until after these systems (along with others) became absorbed into the Experimental Computer Programme in 1967 (e.g. Opit and Woodroffe, 1970, p.80). With the introduction of the NHS Programme healthcare computer systems became directly the prerogative of the Department of Health and Social Security (DHSS) with the regional health authorities (RHAs) taking the responsibility for their development, implementation and evaluation in conjunction with the computer company ICL which was effectively had the monopoly over computer systems for the NHS at the time (Scrivens, 1985, pp.9-10).

Stage 2: NHS experimental computer programme: The technological fix: The first attempt in Britain to develop an integrated strategy on the development of computer systems within the NHS was the setting up of the NHS Experimental Computer Programme in 1967 funded by the Department of Health and Social Security (DHSS) which was intended to cover both administrative and clinical systems. The initiative was the outcome of a report of a Ministry of Health study group set up in 1956 (Barber and

Abbott, 1972, p.3) and started with the DHSS inviting those hospitals where computer systems had already been developed (and the personnel involved) to participate in the programme (e.g. Barber and Abbott, 1972, pp.4 and 89). Fifteen main computer projects were established (later to become fourteen) plus some smaller scientific and clinical ones (Gedrych, 1970; DHSS, 1977; Scrivens, 1985, p.6).

It was originally intended by the authors of the 'Programme' that the systems would be, following evaluation, rapidly implemented throughout the NHS but this did not happen. The general objective was to save much duplication of resources and effort. In this respect the experimental programme can reasonably be viewed a failure. The basic approach was inappropriate for the development and evaluation of computing within the NHS. This was because the rationale for the programme had been inadequately thought out and the technology evolved at a faster rate than the pace of the programme (Scrivens, 1985, p.11). The general assumption was that computers would be good for the NHS although there was little attempt to identify in any detail how this might be brought about (Caddick and Lee, 1974, pp.39-44; Hanby, 1974, pp.79-83; Scrivens, 1985, pp.5-6). This apparent naiveté related, in all probability, to the more general concern of the Wilson government to protect and nurture the British computer industry (Hills, 1984, pp.153-66). This led specifically, to the decision to standardize on ICL mainframe computer systems in 1971 (Caddick and Lee, 1974, p.43). In the words of Mike Healey (London School of Hygiene) a member of the DHSS Research and Development Committee, 'The Americans had the space programme. Britain had ... the NHS ...' (quoted in Laurance, 1981, p.25). What he meant by this was that computer systems were being developed within the NHS less to improve the efficacy of the service and more to support the British computer industry. The experimental programme provided a 'test bench' for ICL computer systems where they would extensively evaluated just as any other form of 'high technology development' within the NHS (Scrivens, 1985, p.6). But because the programme was so highly centralized this led to a great deal of inflexibility being built into the system. There are further parallels here with the American space programme. Not the Apollo Programme of the 'space race' but the more recent Space Shuttle Programme that has also been analyzed as being an expensive, inflexible and unable to provide the service intended (Colleridge, 1990).

Within the programme there was a general belief that the development of computer based-medical records should be a major objective because these would then function both as the point of integration for the hospital systems and helps ensures the active involvement of medical and nursing staff (Gedrych, 1970, pp.345 and 347; Lamb, 1973, p.29). Nevertheless, despite this general belief automated medical records systems never did materialise or more accurately work started but was never completed. To illustrate, work started just such a development at the North Staffordshire Hospital Centre one of the key players in the overall programme. The rationale for the work can be summed up by following quote from a symposium on the project held in April 1975:

> The [computer] network from a medical point of view is incomplete because it does not contain the medical identity of the patient, i.e. the diagnosis, treatment and history. The next step, therefore is to provide a method of holding and presenting that medical information and making it available through the communications network to those who need it in all parts of the system ... [T]his part of the system is currently at the programming stage.' (Smith and Hutchinson, 1975, p.7)

This extension to the system was clearly at an advanced stage of development yet two years later when the DHSS (1977) 'Interim Report' was published the specific system is not mentioned. Nevertheless, automated medical records were recognised within the report as a good thing (like 'motherhood') because they would provide accurate, complete, legible, up-to-date and consistent patient information that was more readily available than the manual system. Only the Queen Elizabeth Hospital in Birmingham, however, was anywhere near being able to provide such a system. The report describes the system there as follows:

> On patient admission, the medical records department prints a multi-part set of documents, each headed with clear, consistent, computer-produced details, and serving the following purposes: Ward Admission Sheet; Diagnostic Summary ... ; 3 History sheets; Nursing record; Operation Record and Anaesthetic Record. (Para. 4.2.3.3.1)

This was not a fully automated system but would have led to medical information being available on the computer system as well as the paper-based medical records folders. Ultimately, however, the belief that patient data and information could be fully integrated within an automated medical record proved to be too complicated and expensive to be a realisable objective within the programme.

It was not, however, simply a matter of technical complexity and costs for the approach to automated medical records systems also failed to take into account that there were, to quote Bittner and Garfinkel (1984), 'organizational reasons for "bad" clinic records'. The argument implied here is that the different stakeholders in the medical record (especially doctors and managers) have conflicting interests in its usage. It is a rationale based on the irreducibility of medical and managerial matters to one common system. The medical profession in the UK has always been very keen to keep the two activities separate in large part to prevent managerial priorities directly impinging on clinical work (see also Chapter 5). It is true that more recently, since the introduction of resource management and the 'internal market', there have been some significant changes with some hospital consultants taking on the role of clinical directors managing departments (see Chapter 7) but that was not the case in the late 1960s and 1970s. That is not to say there were not policies in place aimed at bringing about such a change. The Ministry of Health was very keen to involve doctors in management and set up a working party on the organization of medical work in hospitals together with the Joint Consultants Committee in 1966. The reports, known as 'Cogwheel' (because of the design on their covers) recommended the establishment of medical divisions which would 'promote efficiency in the organization of medical work' (Goldsmith and Mason, 1974: ii). The original reports were published in 1967 but their impact on the doctors was limited. In the third report (Goldsmith and Mason, 1974), which was published several years later, the stated purpose was 'to gain more insight into the reason why divisions had been *slow in tackling many of the problems assigned to them* and the part which the presence or absences of information ... had played in this' (ibid., p.1, *emphases added*). This lack of success was also commented on in the Report on Management Arrangements in the NHS (DHSS, 1972, para. 3.34) where it was noted that 'information is sometimes unreliable, of doubtful relevance and out of date and there are gaps in what is available'. The Experimental Computer Programme was to prove to be no more successful in this area than this other organizational change.

The programme failed to create systems that doctors wanted to use. Initially, it looked as if the programme might deliver automated and integrated medical records systems this possibility soon faded. Neither the systems nor the doctors were flexible enough for it to become a reality. The original 'experimental' approach quietly gave way to a more pragmatic approach in which the various hospital functions were treated independently. Laboratory analysis, for example, would be computerized, but the results would still be printed or written on paper slips and delivered by hand to the relevant ward or clinic.

The situation with nursing systems was not dissimilar. There was work carried out on the development of a real-time nursing record system. But this only took place on one ward at the Royal Devon and Exeter hospital and on three wards at the Queen Elizabeth Hospital, Birmingham (DHSS, 1977, para.4.4.3.1.). Two other hospitals - Addenbrooke's and Charing Cross - were then developing nursing dependency systems (ibid., para.4.4.3.2.2). Six hospitals were at that time developing nurse management systems (DHSS, 1977, p.12 and paras.4.4.1-4.4.4.3). In part this greater emphasis on nursing management was because such systems were technically easier to design and evaluate than the case with systems intended to directly improve nursing care. In this connection the interim report made an insightful remark at the end of the following comment:

> [E]ffort should be expended in into trying to correlate improvements in information with corresponding improvements in patient care in order that the true impact of these systems can be gauged. *Whether*

this can be done objectively remains to be seen. (ibid. para.4.4.4.3, *emphases added*)

Nevertheless, it was anticipated that these computer-based nursing records systems would also result in a 'more rational and determinate approach to planning nursing care' (DHSS, 1977, para.4.4.2).

There was a major difference between the medical and nursing systems which related to the capacity of doctors and nurses to influence policy of the programme. In this the doctors played a far more effective role in the actor-network both locally and nationally. Locally, it was often a consultant who 'championed' a project. For example, at the North Staffordshire Hospital Centre this role was filled by Professor Hutchinson a neurologist. It was also the case that the consultants as a group would have to give their support by way of the Medical Executive Committee (e.g. Staffordshire AHA, 1975, p.5). The only representation provided for the nurses was that provided by District Nursing Officer. Nationally, the doctors were strongly represented on the DHSS computer committees as advisers and were (as we shall see) prepared to be vocal in their views. (Laurance, 1981).

Initially the Programme was to have been completed by 1974, but it did not. Its costs, also, rose steeply and this brought it to the critical attention of the Public Accounts Committee in 1976 (Laurance, 1981, p.23; Scrivens, 1985, pp.10-11). The subsequent highly critical report forced a major rethink of the programme's strategy within the DHSS. Subsequently the programme became far less experimental and much more concerned with the development of standardized administrative systems (Scrivens, 1985, pp.9-10). One consequence of this change was a revolt leading to the resignation (in 1980) of nearly half of the DHSS R & D computer committee because of what was claimed to be the inflexibility of the DHSS. The main complaints related to the DHSS's unswerving commitment to (a) ICL systems and (b) the central co-ordination of all computer developments through the NHS (Laurance, 1981; Scrivens, 1985, p.19). The resignations were also related to the belief that 'the DHSS ... did not appreciate that the definition of efficiency was dependent on the purpose of the system' (Scrivens, 1985, p.19). These resignations indicated an underlying rift between those wishing to develop computer systems to underpin effective management of the NHS and those who were more interested in the development of systems for clinical purposes. One committee that did survive was the Computer Policy Committee. Later, in 1985, it was combined with the Steering Group on Health Services Information (commonly known within the NHS as the 'Körner Committee') to form the Information Advisory Group (BJHC, 1985a, pp.7-9; 1985b, p.8). This group reported to the then newly created NHS Management Board. (Scrivens, 1985, pp.33-4). By that time computer policies were firmly subordinated to the demands of information management (See also Chapter 4). Back in 1976, however, it was the technology that still held centre stage although this was soon to change.

The Computer Programme officially ended in 1981 and with it the DHSS funding (DHSS, 1982, p.1) although to all practical purposes it was already finished by March 1978 (Scrivens, 1985, p.11). The longevity of the programme, however, had the paradoxical effect of inhibiting the diffusion of IT throughout the of the hospital service. The experimental sites monopolized all the available computer resources and the attention of the computer specialists located within the headquarters of the various Regional authorities (Scrivens, 1985, p.17). With the demise of the programme these specialists had to look for new projects if they were to retain employment within the NHS in the 1980s and beyond. It is to this story we now turn.

Stage 3: Corporate systems: From technology to information It was in 1980 that the Joint NHS/DHSS Steering Group (chaired by Edith Körner) was set up. This committee was to have radical implications for computer policy within the NHS. Its remit was to look at the management information requirements of the NHS and make recommendations (Mason, 1984, p.24) - including clinical information (NHS/DHSS, 1982a) the traditional province of doctors. The recommendations of the Steering Group were made mandatory in April 1984 following the introduction of the Griffiths' management reforms (1983) (BJHC, 1984, p.5). It was recognised by the Steering Group and the Department of Health (DoH) that these new information requirements, even though they were minimal, would necessitate new investment in computer systems as most districts lacked the necessary IT. The date for the implementation of most of the committee's recommendations was to be April 1987 (ibid.) and meeting this deadline was an important political requirement fed down from ministers to regional chair(wo)men and general managers. At the time peoples' jobs were seen to be on the line.

The Regional computer specialists were sought to provide a new generation of computer systems that would support these new and emergent management information systems (MIS). If their strategy had been successful they might have been able to retain their central role within NHS computer services. In the event they did not. First, senior management within many of the regions organized the Inter-Regional Consortium (IRC) to replace of the national DHSS funded computer programme. This consortium only comprised the West Midlands, Northern, South East and North West Thames Regions with ICL. Yorkshire and Wales were associate members of the group. Second, the IRC would provide the corporate systems that would provide the computer support for general management. There were four systems being developed and these were as follows:

1. Patient Administration System (PAS)
2. ntegrated Resource Information System (IRIS)
3. Manpower Management System (MMS) [2]
4. Works Information and Management System (WIMS).

They were referred to as the Regional Standard Systems (RSS) and described as '(t)he second generation systems ... designed on a comprehensive view of the information a district needs.' (Abbott, 1985, p.17). In other words, they were to be based on the systems developed at the hospitals that formed the project sites in the experimental computer programme. This strategy reflected a lack of responsiveness to changing requirements of management within the district health authorities and the hospitals. This point is well illustrated in the following case study.

Corporate computer systems: Case study

The research was carried out during 1986 and focused on prospective users' responses to the implementation of three of the corporate systems (PAS, IRIS MMS). The research team consisted of David Cox, Judy David. Ruth Green and myself. We found that the health district managers were generally satisfied with the Patient Administration System (PAS) (Dent et. al., 1992, p.133). It was the one major system to emerge from the experimental computer programme. Its strength lay in its role as an operational system but its vulnerability was its inability to provide management information. The district and hospital managers were far more dissatisfied with the inadequacies of the MMS and the long delays with the implementation of IRIS (Dent et al., 1992). The precursors to the MMS and IRIS systems also lay within the computer programme but these were both non-interactive batch systems centrally located at region headquarters. The earlier version of the MMS was little more than an adjunct to the batch-mode Standard Payroll System (SPS) (NHS/DHSS, 1984, para. 5.2-5.4) as such it was not interactive and was too inflexible to function adequately as a management information system (MIS). Consequently, they all had to be redesigned and extensively (re)programmed. If the computer specialists failed to deliver the 'new' systems within the time scale their future within the NHS would be in serious doubt. Not that this was the only consideration in determining the future of these specialists (See Chapter 4).

The MMS ('workforce') system was to have been implemented 'module' by 'module' in one region during 1986 so that it might be sufficiently complete to meet the requirements of the Körner report by the April 1987 (the government's deadline for their implementation) (BJHC, 1984, p.5). IRIS, by contrast, had experienced problems at its pilot stage and its implementation was, as a result, delayed for more than twelve months well beyond the 'Körner' deadline. Paradoxically IRIS did get to be fully implemented while MMS was eventually abandoned as one of the IRC corporate systems (Interviews, 1989).[3] The problem for the designers of MMS was that while they able to have modules operational by the deadline the system was of very limited use and its data was unreliable. In important part this was a consequence of it sharing a common coding system provided from within IRIS. Without IRIS in place MMS data could not be relied on. In consequence, managers preferred to rely on their own manual records and treated the MMS system as an added burden requiring data-input but unable to provide much in the way of useful information. In the end, as might be expected, it was the acceptability and usability of the systems that dictated their survival not whether they met the deadline.

In the rational terms of a systems logic, the haste to implement the MMS system did not make sense. It would have been better to have implemented the IRIS system first and then complete the development of the MMS system based on an agreed coding system. This logic, however, overlooks politics of the situation. The regional management services and computer specialists were more vulnerable over the MMS system than IRIS. The accountants were committed to the new system. They saw it as a 'real-time' improvement on the previous 'batch' system and were prepared to accept the delay in order to get what they wanted. The personnel officers were, by contrast, less committed to the MMS system largely because the facilities offered were of unproven worth. Yet unless the Regional computer specialists took the initiative to rapidly develop a workforce system (i.e. MMS) the concept of an 'in-house' integrated corporate system (providing financial, patient activity and human resource data) could not be sustained. In order to reinforce this corporatism (and with it the interests of the regional computer specialists) the development and implementation of all the corporate systems was funded out of moneys 'top-sliced' from all districts' budgets. The systems were offered to the district authorities at discounts, initially of 50 per cent but when this proved to be an insufficient incentive it rose in some cases to 100 per cent (Dent et al., 1992, p.129). This discounting was not always seen in a positive light by district management and the corporate systems strategy became a contested issue between the different levels of management within and between regions and districts (ibid.). Many district managers were aggrieved at having to pay the costs of the computer systems (through the 'top-slicing' mechanism) for, regardless of the reduction in price, it effectively prohibited them from purchasing commercially available systems. (ibid.). This they viewed as an attack on their district's newly emerging autonomy.

While the new information policy presented an opportunity to the regional management services and computer specialists the government's imposition of the April 1987, 'Körner deadline' severely constrained the performance of the corporate systems. These systems were intended to automatically deal with the Körner requirements yet none were ready in time. The introduction of the 'Körner' information systems, coupled with the introduction of general management, provided a prima facie rationale for the Corporate Strategy. In reality, however, they marked its foreclosure for the strategy was insensitive to the concerns and requirements of the health districts. Partly as a response to this perceived over-centralization of computer support some health districts began appointing their own computer specialists. The emergent interest among these district-based groups of computer specialists was the development of computer networks as a putative solution to integrating district health information systems and with them integrative management control. It is to this subject I now turn.

Stage 4: Networking: The technological fix? A network in computing terminology refers to an inter-connected collection of computers and related technologies. More precisely it is a collection of telecommunications equipment and transmission lines used to link computers, terminals, printers, telephones, fax machines, etc. together (Gunton, 1990, p.36). There are three main reasons for organizations adopting this approach:

1. several computers can be linked together to create a more powerful (but flexible) system;

2. users can have a wider range of services than would otherwise be the case;

3. users spread over a wide geographical area can make use of a common system.

There are two general kinds of networks wide area networks (WAN) and local area networks (LAN) but the technicalities involved do not concern us here (see Stokes, 1988a, p.32; Gunton, 1990, pp.110-11 and 199). What is relevant is the role given to IT networks in the wake of the Resource Management Initiative and the re-organizations following the *NHS and Community Care Act* (1990).

During the 1980s to some progress was made in establishing common protocols based on Open Systems Interconnections (OSI) that would enable all types of health care computing systems to be integrated within one or more network(s) (e.g. Stokes, 1988a, pp.32-5; 1988b, pp.140-3; 1989, pp.33-5). The National Strategic Framework promulgated by the NHS Management Board in 1986 called upon each region to 'produce regional information strategies ... ' (BJHC, 1986, p.13). Some regions, including the East Anglian RHA (BJHC, 1987, p.7), committed themselves to region-wide networks whereas others, including the one on which this book is substantially based did not. The role of networks was further reinforced with the publication of the *Working for Patients* White Paper (HMSO, 1989a). In the supporting paper, Review Project 25 on Information (NHS/DoH, 1990, para. 4.9) an IT networking strategy is clearly set out:

> With the envisaged future increase in information flow, automation needs to be examined if the NHS is to avoid the enormous cost of clerical processing. Data communications networks for electronic data transmission can be expected to be of substantial benefit.... The NHS is increasingly using data communications networks and most RHAs have such networks.

This point links directly to the case of resource management. There were two contrasting approaches to networking commonly known in computing circles as *incrementalism* and *Big Bang* and particularly associated, within the NHS, with the initial implementation of the HISS programme (to be discussed later in this chapter). In discussing these two approaches my intention is to explore the tensions between the technical rationality of the computer systems and the social and organizational dynamics as well as any 'unintended consequences'.

Incrementalism largely characterised the IT provision for the Resource Management Initiative (1986). This was largely a pragmatic consequence to the limitations of computer provision at many hospitals rather than reflecting any rejection of a *Big Bang* approach. Most of the original pilot sites adopted some kind of feeder system approach whereby relevant data for resource management was extracted from pre-existing operational systems or adding in additional ad hoc systems as required (Resource Management Directorate, 1989, para. 1.10). The one exception was the Royal Hampshire County Hospital which adopted a more integrated HISS like approach (ibid., 1.11; Packwood et al., 1991, p.44).

The Resource Management Initiative continued from where the Griffiths' Inquiry (1983) left off. In principle the new system of hospital management was to mark the end of medical hegemony. The Griffith's Inquiry (1983) recommended the integration of NHS management into a single line of command. Subsequently doctors did find their influence lessened on formal management boards within districts (Cox, 1991, p.98) but at hospital level their professional dominance hardly waned at all. They also began to successfully compete for the new management posts at that level. By February 1986, 19 per cent of all hospital managers were doctors (Cox, 1991, p.97).

In the wake of the Griffith's reforms came management budgeting, intended among other things to impose budgetary controls on doctors (Preston et al., 1989; Bloomfield et al., 1992, p.204). It was this policy that became (in 1986) transmuted into the Resource Management Initiative (Ham, 1992, p.179; DHSS, 1986, Appendix I, para 1). One important consideration was that 'resource management' was thought to be less provocative than 'management budgeting' to the medical profession. The term 'resource management' was defined by the Resource Management Directorate (January 1989, para 1.2) as a 'hospital management process involving doctors, nurses and other clinical and managerial staff in strategic and operational decision making ... a process underpinned by a patient based information system'. Central to this information system was the 'case-mix management system' (ibid., para. 1.9) which would extract data from the PAS and various departmental systems (see 'Types of computing' above) in order to identify costs associated with each patient. In practice it was the cost for each category of patient that became the goal and hence the average (rather than actual) cost per patient. The system was never intended to provide individualized bills as is the case in the US but, initially, to aid clinical management's review of patient activity and resource allocation (Mountney and Sanderson, 1993b, p.37). Subsequently, with the introduction of the internal market, 'it [became] necessary to develop a tool to enable contracting at a level more sophisticated than block contracts' (ibid., p.37). The basic concept derived from the US system of Diagnosis Related Groups (DRGs) for relating cost and hospital treatment and care (Sharples, 1987, pp.27-31). But because of differences in clinical practice between UK and USA as well as the systems of reimbursement those working at the national level on case-mix decided to design and implement a version of patient groupings to be known as Health Related Groups (HRGs). This is a system designed to identify patient groupings in terms of health need and prognosis (Mountney and Sanderson, 1993b, p.37) based on either the International Classification of Diseases (ICD) (version 10) (NHS Management Executive/IMG News, 1993, p.12) or the Read Code equivalent (version 3) (O'Neil, 1993, pp.22-3). The National Case-mix Office had been established in 1990 and by May 1992 the first version of HRGs was published complete with software package. The system is not yet in routine use within hospitals although at time of writing a complete version has now become available (Research interview, June 1995) and is expected to directly influence contracting from 1995-96 (Mountney and Sanderson, 1993, p.36).

There is much in the resource management that echoes the attempts of the US to implement Utilization Reviews back in the early 1970s (in order to contain the costs of Medicare and Medicaid) and which was eventually replaced by medical audit systems (Chapter 5) because of the unrealistic complexity and expense of the accounting systems (e.g. Freidson, 1976, pp.288-9; McSherry, 1976, pp.123-6). A more recent commentator, namely Wood (1991, pp.27-8), makes the point that developments in utilization review in the 1980s have overcome the earlier problems. Drawing on the work of Ermann (1988) he argues that this has been achieved by focusing 'much more sharply on the appropriateness of treatment' rather than simply the costs. This is because the new generation of reviewers are professional carers (nurses and doctors) and not accountants. This optimism is more than offset, as Wood (1991, p.35) notes, by the fact that the US has been unsuccessful overall in controlling healthcare expenditure. This is largely, he suggests, a consequence of the American public's general preference to trust experts rather than politicians. This experience needs to be borne in mind when assessing the potential effectiveness of resource management and case-mix systems in the UK.

Turning now to the second strategy (*Big Bang*), this characterised the early stages of the Hospital Information Support Systems (HISS) approach. HISS is a derivative of the US acronym HIS or hospital information system (Cross, 1993b, p.39) and was first developed systematically in the El Carmina Hospital in California in the early 1960s (Giebink and Hurst, 1975) and is discussed further in Chapter 5 in relation to medical work. HISS today operates in a way identical to a local area network (LAN) but whereas other

LAN networks are funded out of hospitals' own resources HISS has been substantially subsidized by the Department of Health which committed substantial resources for its implementation (£0.5 billion in England alone) (BJHC, 1989l, p.3).

HISS has been usefully described by the project manager at the Greenwich site in the following terms: '[HISS systems] ... are intended to provide the information technology infrastructure that will facilitate the transfer of policy into practice and will act as a catalyst for the development of resource management and medical audit' (Eames, 1989, p.9). As such, the strategy has all the appearance of being a 'technological fix'. Moreover, in terms of its intended rapid implementation is an example of a *Big Bang* approach (Cross, 1993b). This contrasts with the more 'culturalist' approach adopted within the Resource Management Initiative (RMI) in which IT was seen as supportive of information systems rather than catalytic. This reflected a broader picture within which the concern was to involve doctors in management. In this context imposing 'top down' centralized IT systems would not seem to be a good idea. The flavour of this concern is captured in the following quote:

> We believe a significant involvement on the part of doctors in the management process is a sine qua non of an effective and responsible health service ... We put this view with some emphasis because ... its importance is by no means totally absorbed or accepted part of the current NHS culture (DHSS, HN [86] 34 [Appendix II] November 1986, para. 6)

It could be that the 'culturalist' strategy was designed by the Resource Management Directorate to appeal to the doctors and nurses while the 'technicist' one of the HISS is a concept that appeals to the technicist politicians, managers and specialists because it appears to offer an immediate technical solution to providing an integrated set of hospital information systems that would provide all the management information that might ever be desired. This overlooks the problems associated with the disruption in the change-over, identifying the direct consequences and assessing the costs and benefits (Keen, 1994, pp.173-4).

In many ways early HISS projects had all the characteristics of heroic medicine and it was not only the hospitals that were being challenged by the projects. The suppliers too found themselves confronted with demands many believed impossible to meet. Thorn EMI's 'Software Science' subsidiary, Bull as well as ICL and Istel were all large companies that withdrew from bidding or declined to bid for the HISS pilot sites' contracts (i.e. Greenwich, Darlington and Nottingham). Their stated reasons centred on their belief that the plans were over-ambitious with unrealistically tight deadlines and insufficient funds available (Computer Weekly, 1990a, p.19). The official expectation was that HISS would cost around £2 million per hospital. Critics reckoned a figure nearer £5 million would be the more accurate (ibid.). In the event the cost ranged between £6 million and £9 million per hospital (Cross, 1993b, p.40). It is hardly surprising, therefore, that by the end of 1991 the NHS Information Management Group had decided that the a more 'incremental' approach to HISS should be attempted (Cross, 1993b, p.44) for it would reduce the immediate costs of implementing the HISS programme at least in the short run. One significant consequence of this shift in policy is that the IRC Patient Administration System (PAS) re-emerged as, potentially, a key component within the strategy. This upgraded ICL PAS system, now known as OPENpas, has become the belated centrepiece of the HISS programme for many hospitals (Cross, 1993b, p.44). ICL no longer has the monopoly within the NHS PAS market and now competes with a range of other companies. The main players in this area are now the following: SMS Clinicom; AT&T Istel Totalcare and South Western region's SWIFT system (Cross, 1994, p.5). There were other big players in the field notably McDonnell Douglas, HBO and the GTE/IBM partnership.These companies were each successful in winning contracts for HISS pilot sites but have failed to win large orders in consequence. GTE/IBM have now stopped promoting its systems in the NHS (ibid.). There is some evidence here that suggests that the dynamics of innovation, market relations and IT strategies have not entirely coincided. How this is to be understood is the question I now turn to.

The *Big Bang* HISS projects coincided with a high point in the promotion of privatization and marketization policies by the Thatcher government. Just as the internal market was introduced with the NHS reforms of the late 1980s (see Chapter 7) so too was the pressure for the marketization of computer systems and services. The HISS strategy created the opportunity for an injection of market competition right into the heart of NHS computing and at the same time finally break the domination of ICL systems and the Regional Computer Centres (RCCs). The transactional costs for HISS and other expensive 'state of the art' programmes, however, are high and the conditions of uncertainty and complexity coupled with the small numbers of suppliers all indicate that the dynamics of market competition would be very much attenuated. It is technically necessary for there to be extensive bureaucratic regulations covering such contracts to ensure that the terms of the contracts are properly enforced. At the same time, within the healthcare computing community or network there has emerged and developed an alternative control system which Ouchi refers to as clan control (1991, pp.250-4) characterised by organic solidarity underpinned by traditions of reciprocity and shared values and beliefs. Powell (1991, p.269) offers a similar extension to Williamson's markets failure model with his addition of 'network' to the 'market' and 'hierarchy' forms of co-ordination. Whereas, clan control is a cultural mechanism internal to the organization networks is the parallel mechanism in inter-organizational relations. In contrast to market relations (which are governed by contracts and price as well as being characterised by a culture of suspicion) networks are governed by principles of reciprocity and underpinned by a culture of interdependence.

Whilst the Ouchi and Powell models offer elegant typologies that is all they are. They are designed to clarify and simplify the complexity of organizational internal and external relations. They can, therefore, only be suggestive of the dynamics of intra- and inter-organizational relations. In order to gain a more detailed understanding of the dynamics of IT strategies it is informative to look to a Foucauldian mode of analysis. This is provided by Bloomfield and Coombs (1992) who have emphasized the disciplinary power content of organizational and occupational cultures in their links with IT systems. They argue, however, it is not the case that only one group dominates but rather there are coalitions (or actor networks) drawn from within management, medicine, nursing and elsewhere. For example, it is not simply a question whether HISS centralizes control or not. Rather it is the role it plays (or does not play) in the changing configuration of the social, political and technical system that constitutes a hospital. The implications of this position are explored in the subsequent chapters.

In relation to the marketization of computer systems and services it was the government's active encouragement of new (to the NHS) computer companies to compete for the HISS contracts that changed the IT discourse and broke with the traditions and culture of healthcare computing. The re-introduction of IRC PAS in its new upgraded OPENpas form is not, however, a return to the *status quo anti* for the HISS programme has had its effect. Whilst it has failed to deliver the technological solution to a fully integrated hospital information support system the expensive experience has begun to change the expectations of hospital managers and healthcare professionals as well as of IT specialists. We now have hospitals pursuing incrementalist strategies to integrated systems based once more around the hospital's PAS system. The end-point may be the same but it will be arrived at via an organic ('culturalist') route of adaptation and modification embodied within the resource management programme rather than the technological route of the HISS programme.

Computer strategies: resumé

None of the official NHS computer and IT strategies succeeded in any well-defined sense. Rather than approach the history of healthcare computing, however, in terms of success or failure it is more useful to look at the processes as Latour (1987) recommends as 'fabrications'. The 'Experimental Computer Programme' gave way to the RSS Corporate Systems and the limitations of the earlier programme became 'redefined' and 'rhetorically' closed (Pinch and Bijker, 1984, 1987). In turn, the corporate systems and the regionally centralized strategy that underpinned it soon proved organizationally impossible to sustain. It then became imperative for the regional managers and computer specialists to redefine the systems yet again if they were to retain any credibility. Official NHS computer and IT systems have never fully stabilized yet they have, from time to time, been able to achieve 'black box' status (see Latour, 1987, 2-3) as in the case of the Patients' Administration System (PAS).

The outcomes of the various policies have been marked by a redefining of the purposes of the systems rather than progressing from simple to complex levels of technological sophistication. As the history has shown, the failure of the original 'experimental' systems related to the mismatch between of the computer systems on the one hand and the institutional arrangements on the other, particularly in relation to the medical records. The doctors, in particular, were unwilling or unable to co-operate fully and this led to a greater emphasis ('redefinition') on administrative systems leaving doctors to develop their own clinical systems in isolation. With the introduction of resource management and linical directorates there was a new attempt to introduce some version of computer-based clinical records but without any serious attempt to grapple with the underlying problems involved. There was, nevertheless, a glimmer of insight in the words of Ian Mills, Finance Director of the NHS when he commented in an article in Public Finance and Accounting (February 1989) that the problems associated with the 'introduc[tion of] management budgeting ... had been significantly underestimated and that an over emphasis on systems had led to a neglect of behaviour and attitudinal considerations' (cited in Preston et al., 1989, p.26). Even so this implicit recognition that computer systems are cultural as well as technological artefacts did not influence the original *Big Bang* implementation of HISS systems with the consequence that the approach had to be 'redefined' into an 'incrementalist' strategy by its apologists in order to avoid failure.

Conclusions

In this history of hospital computing the issue of the diffusion of systems was translated first into the terms of the 'stages of growth' framework but on closer inspection was rejected in favour of a four stage periodization that incorporated the organizational dynamics of social constructionism and actor network theory. By adopting this approach it became possible to relate developments in healthcare computing more directly with other changes within the NHS, notably:

1. The move from consensus to general management and then resource management and clinical directorates.

2. The switch from technology to information policies.

3. The injection of quasi-market principles.

Without consideration of these organizational strategies the fate of NHS computing fails to make any sense. Each of these policy changes impacted directly on the healthcare computing actor networks changing the configuration of interests and thereby the actors (and actants) willing to be allied to the new programme. In the beginnings these networks were largely 'driven' by doctors working with computing specialists but, subsequently, computer strategies have increasingly become defined according to management defined criteria. Nurses' involvement has received less attention but has had a part to play throughout. In the next three chapters the role each of the professional groups has played in the development of hospital computer and IT systems will be examined.

Notes

1. The term 'applications portfolio' refers to the range of 'systems' or 'sub-systems' designed for specific functions or activities available for use within the organization (e.g. accounts, admissions and pharmacy).

2. The term 'manpower' is clearly a misnomer. Nursing, which is by far the largest occupational group employed within the NHS (see Chapter 6), is only about 10 per cent male (Walby et al., 1994, p.67).

3. MMS is still in use in one health authority and probably others too. These will be sites that had agreed to adopt the workforce system prior to the IRC abandoning its development.

4 Computer specialists, 'hybrids' and information management

Introduction

The general question to be addressed in this and the subsequent two chapters is the following. What are the implications of healthcare computing and information technology (IT) for the professions most directly affected? There are three professions to be discussed: computer specialists (Chapter 4), doctors (Chapter 5) and nurses (Chapter 6). The inclusion of doctors and nurses is self-evident for their work is core to the delivery of hospital healthcare. They experience healthcare computing and IT as aids or hindrances to their hospital work but for the computer specialists these technological systems are their work. Does this mean that these specialists therefore have more control or influence over the way that healthcare computing and IT develops than the other professions? In part that question has been answered in Chapter 3 but not in terms of the politics of occupational autonomy and control. These are the issues to be taken up here and which will also serve as a basis of comparison with the different modes of occupational autonomy adopted by the medical and nursing professions.

Computer specialists have been the occupational group responsible for the physical introduction of computer systems into the hospitals as well as providing the technical support. They constitute a profession in as much as there is a fully constituted professional association - the British Computer Society (BCS) - which organizes courses and qualifications for individuals seeking professional status. Unlike medicine and nursing, however, there is no legal compulsion to become formerly accredited nor is state registration required. Computer specialists employed within the NHS were rarely graduate entrants from accredited courses or individual members of the BCS. The general policy was one of 'learning on the job' - it was 'hands on' knowledge of the systems that counted. The consequence of this was that pay rates were not high but the labour turnover was (Kenny, 1974, p. 130). The 'work' and 'market' situations (Lockwood, 1958; Abercrombie and Urry, 1983) of these specialists was very different from those of other professions working within the NHS. Their status and autonomy rested more on the management strategy of *responsible autonomy* than professional autonomy as such (see Chapter 2). It is against this background that two central issues are to be considered. First, what strategies, if any, did these specialists adopt to protect and advance their work autonomy, status and security within the NHS? Second, how far were these strategies successful?

The general argument here will be that the strategic shift in emphasis from 'technology' to 'information' management within the NHS fundamentally challenged the autonomy and control of the computer specialists. In attempting to counter this threat the specialists attempted to re-define their roles and organization within the NHS. It is this story of strategy and counter-strategy that this chapter is most concerned. I begin with a discussion on the changing roles of computer specialists up until the mid 1980s including some details as to what specific occupations are included under the generalized heading of 'computer specialist'.

From the mid 1960s to the mid 1980s were halcyon days for computer specialists. These came to an end in the late 1980s when the policy to privatize computer support services was introduced. Details of these changes are discussed in the second section on 'The changing ecology of IT within the NHS' which also includes a case study of Qa Business Services Ltd. as an early example of privatization. It is against this backcloth of recent history that the issue of 'hybrids' and the emergence of 'information management' within the NHS is discussed and analyzed in the third section. There then follows a brief conclusion summarizing the main characteristics of occupational trajectory of NHS computer specialists and their organization.

The changing roles of the computer specialist

First, it will be useful to clarify what occupations are being referred to here under the rubric of 'computer specialist'. The term is adopted so as to emphasize the computer technology component of their IT work (in contra-distinction to information). Moreover, the occupational title is also a commonly recognised one. A computer specialist is a person who will be engaged in one or more of the following activities: (a) systems analysis and design; (b) programming; (c) team leadership and project management. Data processing and entry related occupations are excluded as these are not specialist roles. It will also help our understanding of the current changes if I sketch in some general history for will help explain why their status and autonomy have been questioned. In the 1970s they were able to command good salaries based on a buoyant labour market and within their employing organization could dictate the form computer systems took. This was a problem for both for management and those who use the systems. Senior management has adopted a range of strategies to attempt to extend their control over the computing while computer specialists have responded by developing their own. This is not to suggest that senior management generally is well informed on matters relating to computing. To quote one observer writing in the *Financial Times* in the late-1980s: 'It is universally acknowledged ... that there is hardly a board [of Directors] in existence which has the necessary skills and experience to make informed decision about IT strategy and spending' (Cane, 1988, cited in Murray and Knights, 1990, p.181). Nevertheless, management writers have taken on the task of advising executives how best to manage their computing resources. Nolan (Gibson and Nolan, 1974), whose views became almost an orthodoxy on this matter, suggested that computing departments be, firstly, be fragmented with small groups of in-house computing specialists being attached to user departments. The intention was to make computer specialists more responsive to the user. Secondly, computing should become organizationally subordinated to an information executive. In general terms this is what has happened within the NHS over the last decade or so. Pettigrew (1974, 1975), aware of such strategies within business generally made a number of suggestions aimed at the computer specialists. Essentially, he argued that in order for them to retain their autonomy they needed to be more responsive to user requirements by restructuring and adopting a more project-based model of working.

It was not simply a matter of organizational politics. Any rationale for the occupational and technological monopoly of centralized computer departments was beginning to be seriously eroded by the mid-1970s. They were economically too expensive and technologically unnecessary. The centralized 'in-house' computer departments producing custom-built systems based on mainframe technology became too expensive in face of cheaper, more flexible and increasingly powerful 'stand-alone' systems and PCs. Similarly, the growth in the availability of good quality software 'packages' was making the users far less dependent on the 'in-house' computer specialists. These changes were slowly to have an impact on the NHS for as elsewhere the computer departments were centralized and remained so until the very end of the 1980s or early 1990s. These departments were also like their counterparts elsewhere in remaining committed to the continued evolution and extension of the mainframe-based systems they had worked with over many years. Early use of PC and mini systems within the NHS had been largely restricted to clinical systems (e.g. Dent, 1990a)

When computing was first introduced into the NHS (i.e. Ad hoc stage) computing specialists were mainly programmers who worked alongside keen individuals within hospitals. Probably all computer initiatives in the early phase were the consequence of an individual championing the cause of health care computing and typically this role was one adopted by particular hospital consultants. One such *aficionado* was Professor Anderson, at Kings College Hospital Medical School who attempted to introduce an inpatient clinical records system in the mid-1960s (Opit and Woodroffe, 1970; The Times, 1982, p.13). Another was Professor E. C. Hutchinson at the North Staffordshire Hospital Centre. The advocacy of Anderson led to an expensive clinical system that ultimately attracted criticism from the Public Accounts Committee on grounds of costs (referred to in the previous chapter). The project at North Staffordshire, by contrast, developed into one half of the widely used NHS Patient Administration System (the other half was developed at the Queen Elizabeth Hospital Centre at Birmingham).

Following the inception of the Experimental Computer Project in 1967 virtually all funding came from the Department of Health and Social Security (DHSS) and computer projects were '... controlled by the regional management services rather than computing specialists ...' (Scrivens, 1985, p.9-10) an arrangement intended to ensure effective managerial control over computing. The arrangement reflected common practice in industry and involved outside specialists in the evaluation of new systems. This typically involved operational research (e.g. Barber and Abbott, 1972, p.84-7) and scientific management techniques generally. Such specialists were also being transmuted into systems analysts responsible for the planning and design stage of systems. In this new role they were intended to be the dominant partners within teams of analysts and programmers. As one systems analyst of the period explained: 'I was an engineer ... joined the [NHS] in 1967 on 'O & M' type work and joined 'computing' as a systems analyst in the early 1970s. I was paired with a programmer' (District Computer Service Manager, 1991). This arrangement reflected the practice in industry generally. The intention was that systems analysts were to function in much the same way as industrial engineers within manufacturing. In the case of computing it would be their responsibility to ensure that the systems were designed and implemented in line with management objectives rather than the possibly esoteric interests of the computer specialists (Pettigrew, 1973a & b). This development has been interpreted by some as the deskilling of computer programming (Greenbaum, 1976; Kraft, 1979; Newman and Rosenburg, 1985, p.394-5). The new occupation of systems analysis did not remain a simple tool of management for very long, however, and soon developed its own knowledge-base (of 'analysis') and with that their own relative autonomy and quickly matured as a fully fledged computer specialism alongside programming within the organized profession (Dickson and Wetherbe, 1985, p.58; Armstrong, 1984, p.115-16).

A threat of deskilling to programmers was also posed by later technical developments (Friedman with Cornford, 1989, p.356-9) and programming today has become largely a standardized and fragmented set of tasks. Moreover, following the introduction of micro and mini systems came pre-packaged software to support these systems. This development went a long way to undermine the need for 'in-house' programmers. Where large scale programming is required, as in the software houses themselves, the division of labour of the programming staff has been rationalized and thereby deskilled (Greenbaum, 1976; Kraft, 1979; Newman and Rosenburg, 1985). In the IBM model, an example which has been adopted widely within the industry, there is a nucleus of a chief programmer plus her/his deputy and a documentation librarian. This elite is supported by other programmers carrying out more standardized tasks (Friedman with Cornford, 1989, p.133-4). There are variants to this model but generally software houses will adopt hierarchical structures (Vliet, 1993, p.62-7).

Meanwhile, it is the organizational and user-related problems rather than programming that have increasingly challenged management attempts at comprehensive standardization. Users, whether as individuals or organizations, are increasingly discriminating as to their requirements. This is especially the case with professionals and specialists including hospital doctors and nurses. This is partly because of the greater complexity of their work and partly because they have an authority to be outspoken not commonly shared by routine clerks and manual workers. Changes in government policy during the 1980s fundamentally altered the 'ground rules' of systems development within the NHS and led to a significant restructuring of the organization of computer specialists. It is this development that the next section is principally concerned.

The changing ecology of IT within the NHS: The decline and fall of the regional computer specialists

During the 1980s the computer specialists were increasingly threatened with organizational extinction within the NHS. It was the Regional Computer Centres (RCCs) that, as part of the Regional Management Services Division, had dominated computer developments from the beginning of the Experimental Computer Project (Brown, 1993, p.21) . For the next twenty years or so virtually all computing development within the NHS was controlled by the regional health authorities (RHAs) and funded by DHSS. As pointed out in the previous chapter this etatist rationale was to prove to be a mistake because the technology changed too rapidly for the centralized system to adequately manage. Moreover, the 'corporate' Regional Standard Systems (RSS) were generally too inflexible for the demands being made of them in the late 1980s when the computer specialists within the RCCs were attempting to disseminate their ICL-based systems throughout the NHS hospital service as the computer-base for the new information systems required for Körner data-sets and the Griffith's (1983) hospital management structure. These new demands put considerable strains on the RCCs ability and credibility as the providers of expertise. In the event they did not survive this challenge and by the end of the decade - and in the wake of *Working for Patients* (HMSO, 1989) - the RCCs were privatized or operating as a regional trading agency (Brown, 1993, p.21).

The happenings within the NHS were not unique even if the particular trajectory the computer specialists followed was peculiar to the NHS. There had long been indications within industry generally that the organizational autonomy and influence of computer specialists were likely to be challenged. As early as the mid 1970s Pettigrew (1974, 1975) published advice for staff specialists, including computing personnel, as to how -

organizationally - they might best survive. These articles serve as a useful starting point for the discussion on the decline of NHS computer specialists. The 1975 article ('Strategic Aspects of the Management of Specialist Activity') is of particular interest for the three following reasons:

1 The article is prescient in suggesting the 'mechanics' of the evolution of computer services within large complex organizations including the NHS.

2 The focus of the article was 'the role and credibility problems of specialists ...' (1975, p.5). This was also a source of the hybrid initiative within the computer profession.

3 The underlying model is compatible with the theoretical approach adopted here.

A key element of Pettigrew's (1974, p.27) analysis rests on his conceptualization of power which he views as 'a relational phenomena'. This is very similar to the way power is understood within the actor network perspective (see Chapter 2). In Pettigrew's model (1972, p.1973a), power is a product of actors' relationships but always constrained both by the organizational domain(s) they occupy and the resources they can draw upon. Whilst in these articles the Machiavellian elements central to Latour and Callon (Clegg, 1989, p.202-7) are not mentioned they are, nevertheless, implicit within underlying 'gatekeeper' model presented in his book *The Politics of Organizational Decisionmaking* (1973a) and summarised in the 'Information control as a power resource' article (1972). In both of these an implicit Machiavellianism is clearly present. In the earlier article, Pettigrew (1972, p.188) states, '[p]ower involves the ability of an actor to produce outcomes consonant with his perceived *interests*. The basic units of analysis are not individual persons or groups but *actors* operating from one or more structural positions within a specific social systems' (*emphases added*) which is consistent with the actor-network model. Whilst in his later book (*The Awakening Giant*):(1985) the Machiavellianism is clearly present when he extends his analysis to distinguish between ' a process front stage' decision making and power and 'back stage' structures of control and domination in which managers strive through 'a process of symbol construction and use value ... to create legitimacy for one's actions, ideas and demands, and to delegitimate the demands of one's opponents' (ibid., p.44 cited in Reed, 1992, p.109-10). This is very similar to Pinch and Bijker's (1984) concept of 'rhetorical closure' where members of the core set developing a particular artefact publicly asserts that it works well.

To return, however, to the issues of specialist influence and autonomy, in the 1975 article Pettigrew takes for granted that computer specialists will

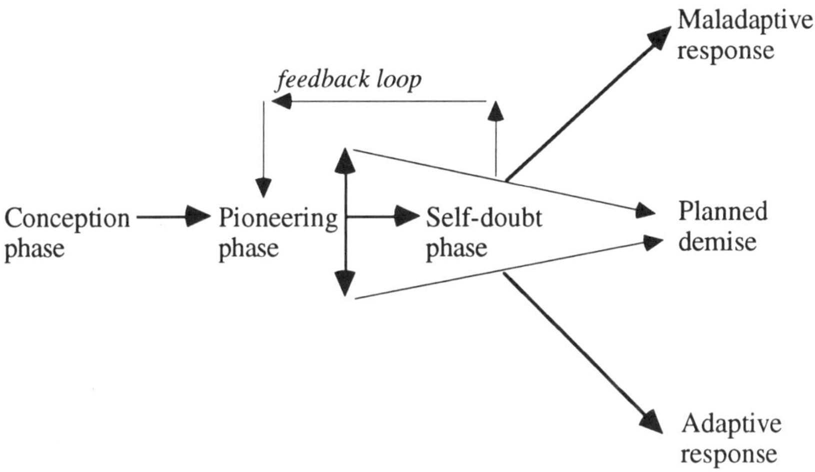

Figure 4.1 Evolutionary phases of computer specialist units

Source: Pettigrew, 1975: 7 (slightly modified)

from time to time have a credibility problem *vis á vis* their clients. In light of this they need, he argues, an effective strategy if they intend, organizationally, to survive. This primarily involves 'an exploration of the political and strategic context of the [computer] specialist's ... work' (1975, p.6). Before continuing any further it will be useful to present Pettigrew's model of the evolutionary phases of specialist units (Figure 4.1). Originally the various stages were of relatively short duration with the 'self doubt phase' coming round about eighteen months after the inception of the department (1975, p.8). This reflected the time between the implementation of the first computer systems and everyone involved having had opportunity to have an opinion on its usefulness. It is also the case that computer specialists are subject to longer phases of 'self doubt' as, for example when they are confronted with major technical and/or organizational changes as, for example, in the case of the introduction of micro-computing and PCs (Burnett and Nolan, 1975). Within the NHS the critical scrutiny of the Public Accounts Committee (PAC) review in 1976 (see Chapter 3) had a precisely such a major impact on the work of the computer specialists. In that instance the NHS computer specialists' response was to move away from innovation and experimental clinical systems and wed themselves even more strongly to the centralized and standardized administrative systems. This is represented by the 'feed-back loop' to the 'pioneering phase' in Figure 4.1. Then came the realisation among many managers (in the 1980s) that the standardized administrative systems were unable to adequately support the post-Griffith's management information systems. By then, however, it was too late for the computer specialists to adequately redesign the systems or introduce new ones. In the end, the computer specialists had their demise planned for them. The NHS Management Executive came under government pressure in the late 1980s to let market forces intervene. Under the new order the NHS had to 'contract out' all 'non-core activity' defined to include the RCCs. In the intervening period some individual computer specialists were appointed as computer services managers or similar within the district health authorities (DHA) (Dent, 1991, p.349) but this was not an option open to most members of the RCCs. More than half the RCCs are now owned by companies such as Sema, AT&TIstel and Anderson's and the remainder operate as regional trading agencies or similar within the NHS (Brown, 1993, p.21).

The move from 'hierarchy' to 'market' - to paraphrase Williamson (1975) - was to prove a very difficult period for most of those involved and particularly so for those who played a significant role in the DHSS computer programme. To explain why this might be so I will now turn to the case of the West Midlands RCC. It became something of a *cause célèbre* and represents a failed strategy to preserve a future for the NHS computer specialists within the new and increasingly hostile environment of the internal market. The strategy married the interests of the computer specialists and the ICL Patient Administration System that had been the mainstay of the specialists' work for more or less fifteen years. It was perceived by many as the 'backbone' of any hospital system and likely to be in demand for the foreseeable future. An Inter-Regional Consortium (IRC) of NHS regions and ICL had been set up in 1985 to upgrade the PAS system to meet the Körner requirements for basic data (BJHC, 1985c). Membership comprised of West Midlands, Northern, South East and North West Thames RHAs (Yorkshire and Wales were associated members). At that time each region was to contribute £200,000 per annum to fund the project. Senior managers from the West Midlands RHA were to chair the management board and committee (ibid.). A modified PAS system - complete with a District (patient) Information System (DIS) - was intended for full implementation by April 1987 (ibid.). While the new operational system was completed the district information system was not. In December 1988 the BJHC (1988a, p.3) reported that there was some 'dissatisfaction' which 'centre[d] on DIS...'. This was probably the last software development embarked on by the consortium for by 1989 events rapidly began to outstrip the RCCs ability to adapt. The publication of the NHS White Paper (HMSO, 1989a) made it clear that the future organization of the NHS would be unconvivial for corporate bodies like the IRC. The Department of Health (DoH) sent out a confidential draft circular (ref. HC89/HNFP89) outlining the 'new roles for regions, districts... and special health authorities based around core activities..' (BJHC, 1989a, p.5) and in future the core activities of RHAs would not include computer services. This circular was swiftly followed by a letter (dated 22 March 1989) from Duncan Nicholls (then chief executive of the NHS Management Board) to all regional and district general managers, stating that RHAs had to review all their services. Moreover, this review had to consider 'whether the services need to be provided at all... [and] whether more effective means exist for their provision than managing them on the traditional model within an RHA structure (cited in BJHC, 1989b). The process of review was to be relatively rapid. 'Broad brush' submissions from regions were required by the 5 May (less than two months later) and fully worked up proposals after six months (30 September). Any services retained would have to be 'demonstrably managed on business-like lines' (ibid.). For the computer specialists within the NHS the future looked most uncertain.

An early victim of this radical reorganization was the management services division of the West Midlands RHA which included 'UK's largest health computer systems development team' (BJHC, 1989c). This division became subject to a management 'buy-out' in December 1988. The sale was agreed in the summer and completed by the October 1989 (BJHC, 1989d). The management team at that time were hopeful that there would be private sector companies keen to enter the health care IT sector and, therefore, be interested in 'buying [the] team' (BJHC, 1989c). In the event only one company indicated an interest and that was the American health IT specialists HBO looking for a means of entering the UK market (BJHC, 1989d; 1989e). The RCC became a private company, in December 1989, under the name Qa Business Services Ltd. It was the first and only IT management 'buy-out' in the NHS (BJHC, 1989f). Initially it looked as if the company would achieve viability if for, no other reason, they expected to be contracted, by the IRC to upgrade the PAS system (BJHC, 1989g) even though the hoped for 'take over' by HBO was to come to nought before the year was out (BJHC, 1989h). The new Qa Business Services Ltd., however, suffered a severe set-back early on when it failed to win the large facilities management (FM) contract with the North Staffordshire HA (BJHC, 1990b). The contract was awarded instead went to Hoskyns, the largest FM contractor in the UK. The company had a 'turnover' of £189 million in 1989 of which FM contracts contributed 47% (BJHC, 1990c). To borrow a football metaphor, Qa and Hoskyns were in completely different leagues. The contract itself was only for low level operational support and the '[a]round a dozen staff' (BJHC, 1990d) previously employed by the RCC cum Qa were re-employed by the Hoskyns.

Despite these disappointments Qa still seemed to have a future. The more interesting and profitable work of upgrading the corporate PAS system remained 'promised' to Qa by the IRC consortium even though, significantly, no contract had been signed (ibid.). Nevertheless, in preparation for this work the new company decided to replace DIS with an Oracle unit (e.g. hospital) management information system designed to 'enable PAS users to progress to case mix, resource management and ultimately HISS' (BJHC,

1990e). This strategy involved adopting a flexible Unix-based approach[1] in the belief that this was what was needed to match the requirements of the new NHS organizational arrangements (especially resource management) (BJHC, 1991b). At the same time as Qa was getting prepared for the new work the IRC was being 'wound up'. It too could not be claimed to be a 'core activity' of the RHAs. At first, this appeared to present Qa with a real opportunity to underpin its future by taking over completely the development of the IRC PAS system (BJHC, 1991a and b). There were, however, complications. To start with the IRC PAS system was Crown Copyright and therefore could not be simply passed from the consortium to the new company without explicit government approval. Nevertheless, according to a spokesperson at the time, the DoH would have been happy to licence Qa as the developer of the system if the IRC could agree and if the users' needs were met (BJHC, 1991b). A consensus within the IRC, however, was not to prove possible because ICL (who was also a member of the IRC) claimed the 'intellectual property' rights on the software and wanted to continue to develop it for their mainframe systems (BJHC, 1991a). In the end all Qa was able to gain any control over at all was responsibility for the support and maintenance of the PAS system (BJHC, 1991b). By October 1991, ICL had been awarded the rights to the future development of PAS (BJHC, 1991c). This turn of events, however, also reflected concerns within the NHS about the future of Qa as it 'had ... publish[ed] disastrous financial results' (ibid.). Moreover, the quality of its work was subject to 'widespread' criticism. A recent PAS upgrade apparently proved difficult to install because of the number of 'bugs' it contained (ibid.). In the words of the secretary to the IRC: 'The ... software written by Qa was an unmitigated disaster' (BJHC, 1991d). The company was now on the brink of going into receivership and its only effective option was to be 'taken over' by one of the bigger players in the market. Unfortunately for Qa the only publicly acknowledged bid, from AT&T Istel, was withdrawn when the news of the loss of the PAS development contract to ICL became public (BJHC, 1991c). In November 1991, it was reported that Qa had collapsed (BJHC, 1991d, p.2).

Just over two years later ICL was awarded an exclusive 25 year licence by the DoH (BJHC & IM, 1994a) this was extremely helpful to them for their market share in health care computing had dropped to around 20 per cent - and looked as if it was going to stabilize at about that figure for the foreseeable future (BJHC & IM, 1994b). This new version of PAS known as OPENpas was to be marketed as part of an incremental HISS strategy (see Chapter 3) with an Oracle relational data-base a strategy very similar to that of Qa three years earlier. Whether ICL would be able to again dominate the healthcare computing market, however, seemed doubtful for new players had successfully entered the health care computing market-place with the top four controlling around 45 per cent of that market (BJHC & IM, 1994b).

It is difficult to know with any certainty what were the motivations of the prime movers in the setting up of Qa. Conversations with some of the people involved in 1989 made it clear to me that several of those in middle-management positions did not view the prospect of the management 'buy-out' as an unmitigated opportunity. The reality was that unless the West Midlands Management Service Division transmuted itself into a private sector organization it would cease to exist creating major problems for computer specialists and others employed within it. It was the case, however, that the 'buy-out' also provided the West Midlands RHA and the IRC consortium with a private sector agency familiar with their general approach to computer systems developments. In the event, market competition prevented the 'business as usual' arrangement from being established. The NHS health market simply became too competitive for ICL even consider allowing Qa to have the licence (and therefore the monopoly) on software developments for the PAS system. Yet without it, and in light of other disappointments, Qa could not commercially survive.

In terms of Callon's categorization this was an attempt at *problematization* that failed (1986, p.196). Qa managers attempted to make the company indispensable to the NHS. The actors, however, wrongly assumed a producer-driven discourse of the kind that had always previously existed in NHS computing. Instead a market oriented discourse was emerging for which the parties appeared ill-prepared. The main issue revolved around the provision of the future software for the ubiquitous IRC PAS system. The failure of Qa to win the contract was related to their lack of success at *intéressement* (or 'enrolling others to their cause') (ibid.). This related directly to ICL viewing Qa as a threat to its own strategy for the post-White Paper era and its keenness to undermine Qa management's attempts to present the company as a useful partner to computer companies wishing to enter the UK health computing market. This particular configuration of actors and actant made *enrolment* and *mobilization* difficult for the new company. Qa's main objective was to enrol the West Midlands RHA and the IRC PAS system into their network along with certain commercial players new to the market but were prevented from doing so by ICL's counter-strategy to protect their threatened and diminishing market share. Without the rights to the software development of the IRC PAS Qa's position was simply one of offering a low cost service to NHS and extensive NHS contacts for new players. It became the a pawn in the competing game plans of the West Midlands RHA, IRC, ICL and the DoH. This is not to suggest a well worked out conspiracy but rather to argue that Qa unwittingly provided the 'rhetorical closure' to the corporate stage of the PAS system. Moreover, the setting up of Qa meant that the NHS managers could begin to adapt to the organizational arrangements without having to concern themselves with the need for a redundancy programme for computer specialists or any consequent industrial relations conflict.

	User Domain	Hybrid Domain	Specialist Domain
Doing Domain	Users	Intermediaries Leaders	Professionals
Driving Domain	Functional Managers	Champions Impresarios	Technical Managers

Figure 4.2 Information systems roles and domains

Based on M. J. Earl 1989

The fate of the other regional computer centres

While the Qa debacle was peculiar to the West Midlands Region all regional general managers had the same problem of what to do about their computer specialist staff following the Government's adoption of a policy of 'privatization, contracting out and the formation of autonomous agencies for anything other than core activities' (BJHC, 1989a). Wessex was the only other region to follow a strategy similar to that of the West Midlands RHA. They set up the Wessex Integrated Systems Ltd (WISL) in a move 'designed to combat problems resulting from a shortage of skilled staff needed to implement its information systems strategy' (BJHC, 1988b). Despite their different approach Wessex regional managers too suffered much public criticism for their inadequate control systems and conflicts of interests (in contracting between the region and the company) resulting from the 'top down' approach to IT strategy and its reluctance to adapt to the new market and information-led approaches (Warren, 1992, p.9).

With the abandonment of the corporate systems strategy the RCCs found themselves confronted with the challenge of 'flexible specialisation' (Piore and Sabel, 1984) with themselves being systematically 'contracted out' of the host organization. In place of the computer specialists came the information specialists. While it was far from essential that this new function be staffed by computer specialists it did provide an opportunity for some so long as they were able to enrol themselves into the newer 'hybrid' domain of information management and technology. It is to this newer actor network that I now turn.

The rise of information management and the IT 'hybrid'

There are two overlapping but distinct strategies currently being applied within the computer domain within organizations. One developed for senior management the other for the organized computer profession. The first is the growth of 'information management' the other, the emergence of the 'hybrid' manager or specialist. In many respects these are different responses to the same pressures and reflect obverse sides of the politics of organizational and occupational control. In computing 'hybrids' have emerged to replace the rhetoric of the 'business analyst' who, with their knowledge of business as well as computing, could act as a 'go-between' between computer specialists and users. With the 'break up' of the large centralized computer departments, however, this intermediary role no longer makes any sense even if problems of communications remain. Rather than identifying new types of roles Earl (1989) suggests that we should view the user and specialist as domains. Moreover, these are separated by a hybrid domain that may be occupied by either user or specialist personnel (see Figure 4.2).

It is not only users who can find computing systems complicated managers are often mystified by them too. At the same time, the specialists tend not to have had the business training and experience to be able to adequately give advice (Friedman with Cornford, 1989, p.297-302; Murray and Knights, 1990). Hence, in the Earl model the hybrid domain covers both the operational ('Doing') and the managerial ('Driving') domains (Figure 4.2). This expansion of the hybrid domain represents a reworking of the inter-specialist 'division of labour' one that reflects the emergence of a new generation of inter-managerial and professional competition (Armstrong, 1984; Murray and Knights, 1990). The growth of the 'hybrid' domain has led to a growing concern among computing specialists as to how they should respond as a profession.

The need for some response has been known for some while more than a decade ago Friedman and Greenbaum (1984) international study identified management's general preference for 'renaissance people' (a poetical term for 'hybrids'). Renaissance people/'hybrids' here refer to computer generalists who have knowledge and experience of business and are able to manage and/or support 'organizational change through the application of information technology' (British Computer Society, 1990, p.9). The BCS viewed this development, at least officially, very optimistically. They asserted in their report that '[hybrids] are the people who seem able to take the idea of a visionary leader and turn it into a reality with the help of technical specialists and other supporting roles in the organization' (ibid., p.9). In the real world of work, however, there were real problems for computer professionals working in the 'hybrid' domain. These related to the ill-defined and ad hoc character of work within this domain. There have been surveys as well as some qualitative research that clearly demonstrates that for computer specialists a 'hybrid' role may well represent a cul de sac in career terms (Rose, 1991 p.102; Earl and Skyrme, 1992, p.177-9). The problem for career-minded 'hybrids' is that 'general managers only start emerging at the top of the organization having been funnelled for much of their career through a specialisation route' (ibid., p.179) and work within the hybrid domain is not generally recognised as a specialisation.

In practice it is easier for business people rather than computer professionals to become 'hybrids' for the probability is that they would have had exposure to IT as users and the opportunity for involvement in project management (ibid., p.178) and such experience would enhance rather than hinder their careers. This presents a dilemma for the computer profession for if 'hybridization' means the employment of non-specialists (in computer terms) then this has real implications for their future employment prospects. In labour process terms the process would appear to represent a de-skilling of computing work (Braverman, 1984) although in practice it is more a case of multi-skilling - or 'polyvalence' (Child, 1985). Whilst this does mean a diminution in the demand for specific technical knowledge and skills this is offset by the demand for inter-disciplinary knowledge and a wider range of IT skills.

Initially the hybrid domain appeared to the computer profession as a challenge in terms of how they were to colonize the new territory. In this they have failed for it has become institutionalized as a new specialism altogether, known as information management and technology. Organizations (including the NHS) have gone through a process of restructuring computing centres with occupations of systems analysts cum programmers being replaced by information management specialists whose career backgrounds and prospects are quite distinct from their computer specialist counterparts. The next section discusses this new phenomenon within the NHS.

Information systems specialists

The management of computer projects within the NHS was heavily criticized by the National Audit Office in 1990 on the grounds they did not reflect any clear IT strategies and were characterized by weak project management (NAO., 1990; BJHC, 1990f, p.8-9). In a review of projects undertaken between 1980-86 the NAO found that 'typical shortcomings included: incomplete feasibility studies; loose contractual arrangements; inadequate planning; weak control; and an absence of post-implementation reviews' (Quoted in BJHC, 1990f, p.8). An important part of the problem was seen to be lack of skilled IT staff (not computer specialists) (ibid.).

Within the NHS the shift in emphasis from computer to information systems and strategies had begun with the Körner reports (e.g. NHS/DHSS, 1982a and b, 1984) and led to the emergence of a new group of information management and technology specialists organizationally distinct from computer specialists. This change presented the NHS 'house' journal (The British Journal of Healthcare Computing) with a problem that they resolved in March 1993 (Volume 10, Number 2) with the adoption of the subheading of '& Information Management'. The emergence of the new specialism within the NHS has been usefully documented by in an article by Herring (1991). The work and responsibilities of this specialism represents a convergence of 'several previously distinct professions such as computer management, systems analysis, information science, librarianship and management' (ibid., p.144). From his review, Herring, concludes that 'there is overwhelming evidence of a growing demand for information professionals and, in many cases, there is a concurrent demand that these information professionals have a *range* of skills and aptitudes *different from those of the traditional IT person*' (ibid., p.148-9 *some emphases added*). He lists the main characteristics of the 'hybrid manager' (1991, p.147) (derived from the BCS report, 1990) as follows:

1. Business knowledge
2. Organizational-specific knowledge
3. Inter-personal skills
4. Communications skills
5. Cognitive capabilities
6. Personality traits and behaviour

This constitutes a formidable list for many computer specialists who are generally regarded (perhaps unfairly) as 'a good technician but a poor communicator' (ibid., p.146). Thus, while computer specialists may be candidates for the new information management posts it is not necessarily the case that they will be the ones to be appointed. The prospects look even slimmer when one looks at the key responsibilities of information managers within the NHS as identified in a Department of Health report *Training for Information Management Staff* (1990, p.3-4):

1. Develop and implement strategies to provide the information required to support the achievement of the business objectives of the health authority or the hospital.

2. Identify the systems required to meet these information requirements and determine the priorities for their introduction.

3. Specify in detail these systems and to co-ordinate their development or procurement and implementation.

4. Organize and manage the operational support required to maintain the information systems.

5. Provide and manage an information reporting and analysis service to support clinicians, operational managers and general managers.

6. Organize appropriate training and development for non-specialist managers and health professionals in the field of information and computing.

The demand for information specialists required the provision of new inter-disciplinary courses in 'information science, information technology, management, systems analysis, communications, psychology and sociology' (ibid., p.149). There are now diplomas and higher degrees in healthcare information management in at least six universities (Brittain, 1992, p.266) including an MA course and diploma programme in Health Informatics at the University of Manchester (Atkinson and Peel, 1992). In the early 1990s the NHS Management Executive and Training Directorate also established a major information management and technology training programme with an annual budget of around £4.5 million (Brittain, 1992, p.266). Yet, despite these developments, the skill, knowledge and competencies for information work within the NHS remains ill-defined (ibid., p.267). Nevertheless, the NHS Management Executive has thought it appropriate to sponsor the establishment of a new professional association to be known as 'The Association for Information Management and Technology Staff' (AIM & TS) which would be independent of other professional organizations - including the British Computer Society (BJHC & IM, 1993, p.4-5). The initiative was presented by Dr Townsend (NHS Training Director) as 'a foundation stone by which we can raise the level of skill in this area' (ibid., p.4). A comment that highlights the real concern of NHS senior management, namely, that while the information management and technology specialism has been invented the occupational space has yet to be fully occupied by people possessing an appropriate knowledge base and range of skills. Even so the new 'profession' has a significant attraction for management as information specialists have no specific technological or organizational base of their own but are reliant on the sponsorship of senior management. It is their role to ensure the health authority or hospital is provided with an effective information system (as defined by senior management) and that the contracts for computing and computer support services are provided at the intended level of service for the agreed price. According to Brittain (1992, p.264) an information unit in a typical health authority will have three or four qualified information staff, which adds up to around '5725 information jobs' (ibid.). This is in all likelihood an underestimate as virtually all hospital units and trusts will also employ some kind of information specialist for at least some of the time as the demand for effective information systems to underpin their whole range of activities and responsibilities (including resource management, contracting, clinical audit and quality assurance) make it imperative for them to have access to their own information specialists.

Conclusions

The purpose of this chapter has been to examine the organizational and occupational trajectory of computer specialists within the NHS, the relevance of the concept of 'hybrid', and the implication of the emergence of information management. The computer specialists were dominant within the NHS computer systems actor network up until the mid-1980s but with the implementation of the Griffith's Report (1983) and the Körner Committee's recommendations (1982-84) this fundamentally changed and the 'balance of forces' between regional specialists, health authorities and hospitals. The regional computer specialists had increasing difficulties in imposing any 'closure' on their corporate systems and whilst some, notably PAS and IRIS, became generally accepted the regional centres could no longer dominate computing and computer development. In broad terms, there were three 'strands' to subsequent developments. First, the growing commitment to marketization within the service meant the end of the occupational monopoly and the transfer of many software specialists to the private sector (often providing computing services back to the NHS under facilities management (FM) contracts). Second, the few computer specialists (mainly systems analysts and designers) who remained within the NHS were often employed by the health authorities.[2] The third and most influential 'strand', however, has been the emergence of information management. This started as a 'hybrid' role that computer specialists might have colonized. This, however, never happened for it rapidly transformed into a new specialism and management discipline in its own right but one that remains firmly under managerial control.

This chapter demonstrates how the profession of healthcare computing was always vulnerable to management control strategies. NHS management was always keen to find ways of containing the autonomy and costs of these specialists in order to gain - in today's parlance - better 'value for money' . In putting in train a strategy of eroding the *responsible autonomy* of the computer specialists the NHS management did not seek to apply new internal systems of direct control. Instead, following the direction of the UK government, they turned to marketization as a control mechanism. In principle, this 'solution' is also available for the management control of doctors and nurses. Yet, for the time being at least, it is a strategy that has not been adopted. In the next two chapters the reasons for this are explored in relation to medical and nursing computer systems.

Notes

1. Unix is a portable operating system that automatically controls and supervizes the computers, peripherals and the running of programmes. Moreover, being 'portable' means it can run on a wide range and types of computers which, in turn, means that 'users' are not locked into relying on one manufacturer's machines only.

2. There are also central NHS computer agencies (notably the Information Management Group of the NHS Management

Executive) which develop policy and generally give advice to the executive. Some computer specialists have followed career paths into these agencies.

5 Medical computing and professional autonomy

Introduction

Hospital doctors, when they have been interested at all, have generally been concerned with developing computer systems for clinical research purposes (Young et al., 1990, pp.16-21). This research orientation has taken two forms, either a computer system was used to support the data processing requirements of a research project or the computer system itself was the object of the research. The use of computers as a research tool is not my concern here - medical computing in this sense is no different to other forms of academic research. On the other hand, research by doctors on the clinical uses of computers is very much of interest. In this chapter medical computing will be discussed in relation to the issues of medical and clinical autonomy, clinical practice and medical audit. Medical autonomy is the outcome of the doctors dominance within the hospital diversion of labour whereas clinical autonomy refers the discretion (or 'indetermination') of the clinical decision-making process. One doctor, for example, might prescribe drug therapy another will prefer to recommend surgery. According to Tolliday's definition (1978, pp. 41-42) this will not necessary be a case where one doctor is right and another wrong but rather that the complexity of medicine and the variations between of patients and their condition (as well for ethical reasons) all make clinical autonomy functionally necessary. As mentioned before (Chapter 2) this is a little simplistic (although not necessarily untrue) for it ignores the role medical dominance (Freidson, 1970) also plays in reinforcing a doctor's clinical autonomy. It is this latter area of discretion that may be becoming more restricted than before with the introduction of resource management and with it the need to consider cost implications when deciding how best to treat a patient. These issues of autonomies have particular relevance in any discussion of computer systems for doctors.

There are three component parts to the chapter. First, following some basic distinctions in terminology, there will be a discussion of knowledge-

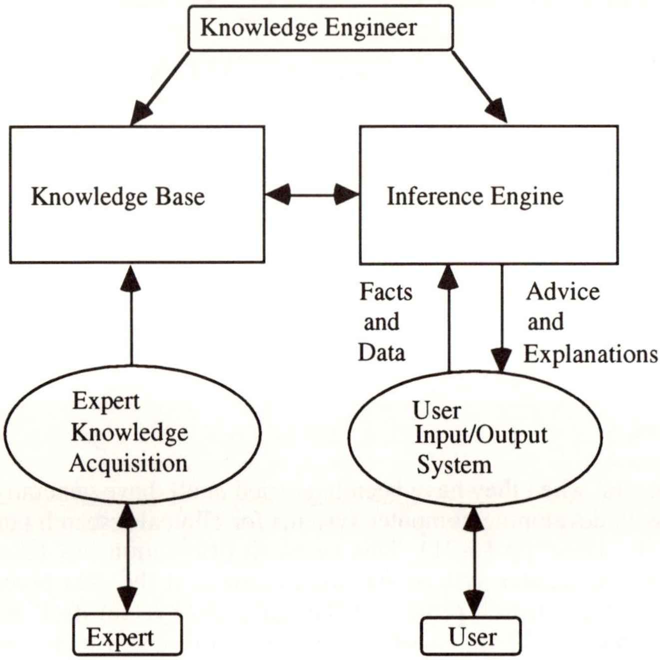

Figure 5.1 Simplified structure of an expert system

based systems and artificial intelligence and their application in medicine. This leads, second, to topic of automated medical records and the doctors' responses. Important considerations here are the issues of clinical and medical autonomy which provide the link to the issue of IT and medical audit which is the third component of the chapter. A central theme will be the issue of automated medical records as this has had a pivotal role in shaping hospital computing. Current developments in document imaging processing (DIP) and clinical workstations which extend the possibilities and applications of automated medical records and clinical records are discussed in Chapter 8. The reason for this is that, unlike the systems examined here, they are either not in general use or there is little research assessment of them available. They are therefore treated as probably characterising the prospects for the immediate future.

The general argument for this chapter will be that medical computing reflects the broader tensions of organizational vs occupational control within the NHS which is reflected in the configuration of the actor networks.

IF the light bulb does not light,

THEN the battery might be flat (Probability 0.2),

OR the connector might not be a conductor (Probability 0.1).

ACTION - Check the battery first!

Figure 5.2 An example of a simple heuristic

(Edwards, 1991, p.47)

Whereas in the earlier stages of healthcare computing doctors were able to dictate the whether and to what extent the systems would be used within the clinic this is now changing. With the introduction of the 'internal market' and resource management systems the emphasis is less on the clinical side of systems and more on the administrative ones of cost and efficiencies. The new generation of systems are intended to integrate medicine more fully into the NHS and thereby subject to greater managerial control. Whether that will be the outcome is still far from clear.

Computing for doctors: data vs knowledge-based systems

It is important to begin by clarifying basic terminology. This is less for the light it will throw on technical matters and more because of the help it provides for assessing the implications it has for medical work. It is the logistics of capturing and storing data that most easily distinguishes data- from knowledge-based systems. Data-base systems are computer 'stores' of data which might, for example, operate as a bed management system or medical record system. A knowledge-base system, by contrast, can offer advice and can give all the appearances of being intelligent. In terms of function, however, data-base medical information systems can provide 'advice', very similar to a knowledge-based system, in the form of 'prompts' for clinical, educational (medical training), or audit purposes. The resources required to ensure that the data-bases are accurate and up-to-date, however, can be very great. Whereas, data-bases are costly and time consuming to maintain knowledge-based systems are not (Szolovits, 1982, pp.2-6; Shortliffe, 1984; Hsu and Kusnan,1989, p.188). This is not to suggest that knowledge-based systems are an easy option for they are not. They require a complex and comprehensive underlying conceptual structure which has the technical ability to emulate human reasoning. Like

IF: 1) THE STAIN OF THE ORGANISM IS GRAM NEGATIVE,
AND

2) THE MORPHOLOGY OF THE ORGANISM IS ROD,
AND

3) THE AEROBICITY OF THE ORGANISM IS UNKNOWN

THEN: THERE IS SUGGESTIVE EVIDENCE (0.6) THAT THE CLASS OF THE ORGANISM IS ENTEROBACTERIACEA

Figure 5.3 A medical example: a MYCIN heuristic

(*Shortliffe, 1976, p.181*)

humans these computer systems have often to carry out reasoning with incomplete information. To do this their designers have provided a system of symbolic reasoning, codified as .i.heuristics; (Shortliffe, 1976, pp.159-94, 219; Fitter and Sime, 1980, pp.60-2) or heuristic knowledge which is the experiential knowledge or the 'art of good guessing' (Feigenbaum and McCorduck, 1984, p.102). To explain, an expert system consists of an inference engine and a knowledge base (see Figure 5.1). The inference engine is the software component that 'drives' the knowledge-base, in other words, it simulates the deductive thought processes of a human expert. A particular kind of systems specialist known as a knowledge engineer will normally elicit the knowledge and experience from an expert or a group of experts and have this programmed as a set of *If* (condition) expressions and *Then* (action) statements. A very simple illustration is set out in Figure 5.2 using the example of an electric torch that does not work. This is followed a by MYCIN example in Figure 5.3 which is structured in precisely the same way, although in this example no 'action' is suggested.

There are other systems that operate as medical decision-aids which also function similarly to knowledge-based systems. There are two that need particular mention here because of their importance in medical computing: the Bayesian approach and neural networks.

The Bayesian approach is not strictly speaking a 'knowledge-based' approach at all. It was first introduced as a technique for medical diagnosis in 1961 and is based on Bayes' theorem. This uses probabilities for determining diagnoses instead of heuristic reasoning Young, 1982, p.1334). This approach offers a very accurate method for calculating the probability of a disease (diagnosis) based on known observations (signs and symptoms). A particularly well known version is the one developed over

**HOW DID YOU DECIDE THAT ORGANISM-1 MIGHT BE E.COLI?

I USED RULE 021 TO CONCLUDE THAT THE IDENTITY OF ORGANISM-1 IS E.COLI.

THIS GAVE A CUMULATIVE CF* OF 0.47.

THEN I USED RULE 084 TO CONCLUDE THAT THE IDENTITY OF ORGANISM-1 IS E.COLI.

THIS GAVE A CUMULATIVE CF OF 0.55.

FINALLY I USED RULE 003 TO CONCLUDE THAT THE IDENTITY OF ORGANISM-1 IS E.COLI.

THIS GAVE A CUMULATIVE CF OF 0.74.

* CF is a measure of confidence of the conclusion being valid

Figure 5.4 MYCIN : sample question and explanation

(*From Davis, Buchanan and Shortliffe, 1977 quoted in Fitter and Sime, 1980, p.57*).

many years (since the 1960s) by de Dombal and colleagues at the University of Leeds to aid the diagnosis of acute abdominal pain and related diseases (de Dombal et al., 1972; de Dombal and Horrocks, 1974; Shortliffe, 1984, pp.53-8; de Dombal, 1991). A DHSS trial in the mid 1980s reported a 65.3 per cent 'initial diagnostic accuracy' for the system as against 45.6 per cent for the doctors (Adams et al., 1986). de Dombal (1991, p.274), who cites the same trial also reports on other studies which provide similar results. There are, nevertheless, problems with the system that relate to the mode of problem formulation and representation of results (Shortliffe, 1984, pp.57-8). Firstly, the system is foreign to the way many clinicians work. Secondly, unlike heuristic approaches (e.g. Figure 5.4), the system is unable to offer an explanation for its advice other than in terms of statistical probability. Nevertheless, the system can be judged a technical success in that it can achieve a distinctly higher level of diagnostic accuracy than previously possible in acute abdominal pain even if its widespread acceptability is likely to be limited.

The second alternative to the heuristic approach is that of artificial neural networks. There has been much interest in this area (Weinberg, N., 1990, pp.155-6) including some within the NHS (Clarkson, 1991, pp.13-14; Yang et al., 1993; Smith, 1994). The first computer science experiments with neural network machines started twenty years ago in England (Weinberg, 1990, p.156). Unlike heuristic knowledge, neural networks are modelled on the topology of the human brain, in particular, its apparent over-provision of interconnections. In other words, they comprise of a mass of interconnections characterised by much duplication, parallelism and connectivity. AI machines based on neural networks are not programmed but learn through sensory input and feedback (Weinberg, 1990, p.156) . These systems appear to have considerable promise and have already been used experimentally for atrial fibrillation in cardiology (Yang et al., 1993) as well as for patient identification and medical record linkage (Smith, 1994, p.195) although they are still in an early stage of development.

Most of these systems (with the exception of the Bayesian approach) raise the issue of whether there is such a phenomenon as artificial intelligence that connects directly with philosophical and ontological questions as to the nature of knowledge and understanding. My standpoint here is that even if such systems were successful in terms of their designer's aims they would not be intelligent in the sense of having understanding. Moreover, while the reasoning programmed into such systems may be analogous to its human counterpart it is not identical to it because a computer cannot suffer emotionally from the results of its own reasoning (Weizenbaum, 1984, pp.202-27; Dreyfus, and Dreyfus, 1989; Jahoda, 1989). This has led Weizenbaum (1984, p.227) to conclude that there is a significant ethical component to the development of artificial intelligence and that we should not allow artificial intelligence to replace human wisdom - although it may well be a very useful aid.

Now that the medical varieties of knowledge-based systems have been presented it is possible to compare the similarities and differences between examples of different types of medical systems. The systems chosen are well-established ones and this means that their strengths and weaknesses can most easily be identified than would be the case if I had selected 'state of the art' systems. Four such systems will be discussed. These will be the knowledge-based systems MYCIN and INTERNIST and the data-based systems PROMIS and COSTAR. This list is a long way from being exhaustive for there are many other knowledge- and data-base medical systems in existence (Giebink and Hurst, 1975; Wardle and Wardle, 1978) and more being developed (Shortliffe and Perreault, 1990). Few, however, have gained the archetypal reputations of these four systems. All the systems appear to have much to offer as electronic aids for doctors that could improve the quality of care they provide their patients.

MYCIN

MYCIN is probably the best known of all the knowledge-based clinical systems ever developed. It is known as a decision support system and was developed by Edward Shortliffe at Stanford University between 1972-78. It is named after a common suffix of many anti-microbial drugs. It was designed to assist doctors to select appropriate antibiotic drugs for patients with serious infectious diseases. The rules were initially acquired from clinical experts but the system also can acquire new rules directly from interaction with a clinical expert (Shortliffe, 1983, p.222). An important characteristic of the system is that it gives reasons for its decisions (see Figure 5.4). Despite its relatively long history the system has not been used routinely in medical practice but continues to be used experimentally and as a teaching aid (ibid.). It has also been used as the basis of other knowledge-based systems in medicine (e.g. PUFF for pulmonary diseases) (Michie and Johnston, 1985, p.42; Hsu and Kusnan, 1989, pp.163-4; Fieschi, 1990, p.220) as well as other disciplines including SACON an expert system for structural analysis in engineering (Feigenbaum and McCorduck, 1984, p.106).

A significant medical successor to MYCIN is ONCOCIN a chemotherapy system developed in the 1980s (Shortliffe, 1986; Sheil, 1989, pp.163-4). What is particularly notable about this system is that it has been designed to work without the need for knowledge engineers. Instead ONCOCIN elicits knowledge via case histories entered directly by doctors onto electronic forms (i.e. screens on the VDU designed to look like paper forms) using keypad and mouse. This mode of eliciting knowledge is made possible by utilising the LISP programme language (because it can handle words and statements) and object-oriented programming (and therefore is focused only on the particular case, Gunton, 1992, p.129). The designers of the system have made the assumption that doctors will prefer to use paper-like records and will avoid using keyboards if at all possible. For this reason ONCOCIN only asks doctors to use a mouse and a numerical keypad.

INTERNIST/CADUCEUS

This system is similar in concept to the MYCIN system. Its knowledge-base reflects 40 years clinical experience of one of its initiators, Dr Jack D. Myers at the University of Pittsburgh (Taylor, 1980, p.256). It too is an experimental programme but in this case it is designed to aid skilled internists in resolving complicated medical problems (Feigenbaum and McCorduck, 1984, pp.87-8; Richman, 1987, p. 52). In contrast to the narrow focus of MYCIN this system covers the broad spectrum of general medicine being more than 80 per cent comprehensive in its coverage of the diseases of internal medicine (ibid.). The system, however, is not without serious deficiencies. These principally relate to the inability of the system to construct diagnoses that span multiple problem areas and to explain the reasons for its conclusions (Barnett, 1982, p.494; Miller et al., 1984, p.203).

A brief excursion

Before moving on to the two examples of the data-base systems it will be useful to pause first to consider why doctors' are resistant to the use of the knowledge-based systems in their clinical work. Yet these systems have long been known to be generally more accurate than real doctors in making diagnoses (Ellison, 1978, pp.30-59; Wardle and Wardle, 1978; Feigenbaum and McCorduck, 1984). Shortliffe (1983, pp.216-17) has suggested the following reasons:

1. Doctors, like other mortals, quickly reject systems that are pedantic in their presentation of knowledge and advice.

2. The correction of errors, or the filling of gaps, in a system's knowledge-base takes time. There is often a delay of months between identifying an error and that error being corrected in the next 'release' of the system.

3. It is an arduous and time consuming task acquiring a knowledge-base, whether based on statistical data or extracting judgmental information from the minds of experts.

To which I would add an important point made by Young (1980, p.522):

4. Diagnosis may not be the most important consideration. Hypertension, arthritis and heart failure, for examples, are all usually treated before the cause (if there is one to be found) is determined. Treatment and views about the prognosis are more important, certainly to the patient.

In any case, computer-based diagnostic (knowledge-based) systems cannot exceed the capabilities of a hospital medical or surgical team as a whole for they are based on the knowledge of real life specialists. In practice, these computer systems have been treated more as research projects than practical clinical tools. A partial exception are those decision systems based on Bayes theorem which will be discussed separately because they are based on different principles and relate to clinical decision-making differently too.

Back on track: PROMIS and COSTAR

In this section I return now to the list of clinical computer systems, this time to discuss the two data-base systems, PROMIS and COSTAR:

PROMIS

PROMIS (Problem-Orientated Medical Information System) is a medical information (data-base) system designed to facilitate the comprehensive and systematic capture of patient information and is based on Dr. L. L. Weed's system of Problem Orientated Medical Records (POMR) (Weed, 1968; McIntyre et al 1972). POMRs does not focus significantly on the identification of a diagnosis. In contrast to conventional approaches it concentrates the doctor's attention on the patient's medical problems and provides a framework for dealing with these systematically over time. To this end the medical record is maintained as a set of active progress notes. The kernel of the PROMIS computer system is a collection of computerized clinical displays called 'frames' which are intended to both guide and teach doctors in their clinical work. These frames are interactive and the doctor can update the information contained within them, while at the same time being guided by 'prompts' the system gives in response to that information. (Giebink and Hurst, 1975, pp.199-200; Willcocks and Mason, 1987, pp.16-17). An important component of the system is the 'audit trail' which is automatically maintained within every patient's file in order to ensure continuity of care/treatment (Giebink and Hurst, 1975, pp.199-200). The system is installed at the University of Vermont Medical Center, Burlington, Vermont where it is claimed to be in operational use in the obstetrics and gynaecology ward (ibid.) but there is little evidence that it has been transferred to any other sites successfully (Fischer et al., 1980).

COSTAR

COSTAR (*COmputer STored Ambulatory Record*) is a medical records system for ambulatory patient care designed and developed at the Massachusetts General Hospital in the USA (Barnett, 1968, Barnett et al., 1979; Young, 1982, p.1335, 1985; Shortliffe and Perreault, 1990, pp.211-14). The system includes modules for dealing with appointments, registration and billing of patients as well as the clinic record. On the clinical side the patient-related data is captured from the doctor hand-written completion of an 'encounter form. Some data is written in by nurses (e.g. height, weight, etc. of patient) and medical secretaries or clerks (e.g. laboratory results). The contents of the encounter form are subsequently entered onto the system by a data-entry clerk or medical secretary.

The patients' records are maintained on computer files which can be produced in any of the following reports:

1. details of the specific medical encounter;
2. a summary (status) report of a patient's medical condition;
3. a flowchart, which displays the temporal course of the disease process, or variations in clinical findings, over time.

These three outputs are produced as printed documents ('hardcopy') for each clinic the patient attends. The data on each patient, and patient group is also directly accessible for statistical analysis in a way that emulates a knowledge-based system. To explain, a consultant may have 'prompts' programmed into the system to remind the junior doctors (or her/himself) what procedures to follow, for instance, when there are complications (Barnett et al., 1978, pp.962-70). The system is technically well developed and its administrative modules have been implemented at a number of sites in the USA and Europe (Fiddleman, 1980). Its clinical facilities have been less widely accepted for reasons which will discussed in the case study that follows. More accurately the system is clinically acceptable only initially after a period of time medical resistance to its clinical use does develop (e.g. Campbell, et al., 1988; O'Dell et al., 1992, p.848).

Data-base systems acceptability

Data-base systems have their problems of acceptability too. These primarily relate the difficulties perceived (by doctors) in incorporating them into the routines of medical work. Thus:

1. Junior doctors learn their clinical skills practising on patients starting with the task of 'clerking' patients on the wards (Rees, 1981). To replace this method with one appropriate for the data capture requirements of a computer system could undermine the training of junior doctors.

2. Consultants, in turn, develop their own, sometimes idiosyncratic, often abbreviated, systems of recording clinical information and resent the imposition of standardized computer systems and are apprehensive of the implications for the management of patients (Young, 1984, pp.663-4; Dent, 1985; O'Dell et al., 1992, p.848).

It is for all these reasons that clinical systems (both knowledge-based and data-based systems) have failed to become widely used. This general medical reluctance to work with such systems was why clinical computing became peripheralized within the NHS Experimental Computer Programme of the 1970s (Chapter 3). Yet the reasons for this reluctance do not appear to be fully appreciated by those introducing resource management particularly where it is associated with a HISS system dependant as they are on the co-operation of the medical staff for capture of up to date and accurate clinical data. This is a little surprising given that the original Hospital Information System (HIS) developed at El Carmino Hospital in California has long been known to have been plagued by low user acceptance, particularly among doctors (Giebink and Hurst, 1975, pp.190-1; Shortliffe, 1976, p.11). Apparently, according to Kaplan, (1982, p.398) the surgeons at the El Carmino Hospital were favourably disposed towards the system because they were generally familiar with (and possibly fascinated by) the technology. It was the internists who objected the strongest to the system on grounds entirely compatible the points already made here, namely, that the system 'constrained and proceduralized the information flow' (ibid.) which in consequence, interfered with their thought processes.

Relatively few computer systems have come to be used routinely as clinical tools for it has only been the committed 'aficionados' who have shown sustained interest in designing and using any of these systems (Friedman and Gustafson, 1977; Anderson and Jay, 1983; Young, 1984). This ad hoc approach to medical computing innovation gave rise to 'a disorganized array of computer languages and computer systems ...' (Friedman and Gustafson, 1976, p.201) with hardly any capable of being transferable from one hospital or clinic to another. There have been some indications that this situation began to change during the 1980s.

There were attempts within the NHS to standardize medical computing on the MUMPS system. This was a combined operating system, high level interpretative programming language and data base management system in the 1970s in order that medical systems might be standardized and thereby transferable from one hospital to another (DHSS 1977, para 5.10.2; West Midlands RHA, 1979). This was the software, for instance, that underpinned the COSTAR system. Whilst proving itself a capable and flexible as well as having official DHSS support this was not to become the path by which transferable clinical systems developed. Instead transferable systems rapidly evolved for particular specialisms which with the sponsorship of particular consultant 'champions' and thereby become the accepted standard. This, for example, happened in the case in renal medicine in the NHS (Will and Selwood, 1985). Similarly, the medical record (Fiddleman, 1980, pp.1-4; Kaplan, 1982, p.400; Shortliffe and Perreault, 1990, pp.211-14). This diffusion of COSTAR is likely to be extended further following a recent report of the Institute of Medicine of the National Academy of Sciences in the United States (Dick and Steen, 1991) encouraging the further development and implementation of computer-based patient record systems. This policy debate is taking place at a time when, as Hausam and Balas (1993, p.649) have indicated the USA is marked by changing regulations, reimbursements' mechanisms and legal environment. In the UK broadly similar political, economic as well as organizational changes would seem to be affecting the development and implementation of computer systems within the NHS. It is to these issues I now turn.

Medical computing and professional autonomy I: Case notes and medical records

During 1994/95 the National Audit Office (NAO) in the UK carried out an investigation of information systems and medical records services (including the case note component) within the NHS (Peel, et al., 1994, p.15). The two reports (Audit Commission, 1995a and 1995b) were published in 1995 under the titles *For Your Information: a study of information management and system in the acute hospital* and *Setting the Records Straight.* Both proved to be damning, although as one pair of commentators perceptively observed 'this could equally well have been (and probably was) said every year for the last 25 years.' (Bywater and Wilkins, 1995, p.10). In the case of information management the general conclusion - as reported in the BJHC & IM (1995, p.4) - was that there is poor management, little real strategy and the investment (on average 1.8 per cent of total hospital revenue) too rarely benefits patient care directly. *Setting the Records Straight* similarly slated the state of the medical records which 'in many cases ... are too fat and badly organized making them difficult to use. Doctors cannot find the information they need to make appropriate decisions about care and treatment' (cited in BJHC & IM, 1995b, p.9). Except for the Tonbridge Report of 1965 this was the first major study of medical records within the NHS. The Tonbridge Report recommendations for standardized documentation were implemented but were never subsequently evaluated (Peel, et al., 1994, p.15). Whilst part of the reason for this was the sheer volume of medical records folders in the system another, I suspect, was probably the politics of professionalism that has long functioned to inhibit the rationalization and computerization of the medical record. It will be this aspect that will form the focus of the discussion here.

The tension between professional autonomy and a state/management defined *responsible autonomy* is clearly discernible within the pages of the medical record. These documents contain information not only for the management of patients but also of hospital resources. The clinical notes' component has commonly been structured in a way that reinforces medical dominance within the hospital clinic and peripheralizes managerial interests. The introduction of computer-based medical record systems threaten to change this balance of forces and thereby undermining the patient-centred rationale of the clinic notes in favour of a more resource management approach. This is clearly demonstrated in the following case study of the introduction of COSTAR at a small hospital in the 1980s. The study reports on events over a decade ago uncluttered by the complications of resource management and the internal market and hence providing a relatively simple and straightforward organizational context within which to study doctors' responses to automated medical records and draw out generalizable conclusions.

Case study: COSTAR, clinic work and case notes

COSTAR was introduced into the outpatients' clinics of St Giles Hospital (not its real name) in 1981 under the leadership of a consultant physician (referred to here as Dr Old) and with the initial support and co-operation of his colleagues. The outpatients' department (OPD) at this hospital was not a large one but it did cover a reasonably wide range of medical and surgical specialities (general medicine, surgery, rheumatology, urology and gynaecology). St Giles was in reality a satellite hospital to the nearby General Hospital. There were eight consultants in all.

A key objective of the system was to replace the hand-written case notes with readily available printed, structured reports, flowcharts and clinical summaries on patients as well as making available facilities for the analysis of aggregate clinical data. The stated objective was to facilitate higher standards of patient care and to stimulate medical research and audit. It was assumed both by the American designers (Barnett et al, 1979, p.1231) and Dr Old that the doctors would prefer to use paper documentation rather than access a computer terminal directly.

It would be impossible to understand the outcome of the computer implementation project without some knowledge of the role played by the medical records in the organization of the clinics. As with any other acute hospital, the OPD served four basic functions:

1. A diagnostic service for general practitioners (GPs).

2 An anteroom to the hospital wards and operating theatres enabling investigations to be carried out without the patient occupying a hospital bed.

3 Monitoring the long-term outcome of major surgery of discharged patients.

4 The long-term medical treatment of chronically ill patients.

Functions' 1. and 2. refer predominantly to 'new' patients, while 3. and 4 relate to 'follow-up' patients. According the an internal report of the time approximately 25 per cent of patients attending the clinics were new patients referred by their GP and there were, on average, 120 patients attending each week: 25 per cent in General Medicine , 17 per cent in General Surgery, 15 per cent for Urology, 43 per cent for Gynaecology. Outpatient consultations lasted on average 23 minutes for all clinics.

There was considerable variation in the organization of the outpatient work reflecting the nature of the specialities and the preferences of the consultants. The usual arrangements (by speciality) were as follows:

1. *Medicine*: There were 3 consultant physicians (rheumatologist, bronchial specialist, general physician). (a) The two specialists shared the services of one SHO. Much of the workload was the care of the long term chronically ill. The SHO functioned as an assistant to the consultants and there was little emphasis on medical training. (b) The general physician was allocated one SHO who would only see new patients in the clinic. It was her (or his) task to 'clerk' them, arrange any investigations and arrive at a preliminary (presumptive) diagnosis

prior to the patient seeing the consultant a week later. Thus, there was a training element similar to that found on the wards (Rees, 1981, pp.56-9).

2. *Urology*: The two consultants shared one SHO. Generally the SHO saw 'follow-up' patients. One of the consultant monitored the work of the SHO by checking what had been written in the case notes and writing the letters to the GPs. It is a routine for doctors to write to GPs following an attendance at clinic but usually the junior doctors write their own.

3. *General surgery*: This clinic functioned very much as an ante-room to the operating theatres and the consultant did not see this as appropriate work for a junior doctor. Routinely patients would also re-attend as 'follow-up' patients following surgery. One reason given for by the consultant for not using junior doctors for outpatients' work was that he personally wished to monitor a particular group of patients who had undergone major treatment for cancer and in whom he had a particular interest.

4. *Gynaecology*: The gynaecology clinics also functioned largely as an anteroom to the operating theatres and wards. There were two consultants involved neither of whom employed SHOs to assist them. One, however, being a senior lecturer at the medical school with academic commitments which at times clashed with the outpatients' clinics often delegated his outpatients' work to a senior registrar assisted by a registrar (or SHO). In addition, medical students would attend these clinics as part of their training.

The COSTAR system was intended to replace the hand-written record and it is only by understanding the actual practices of the doctors will it be possible to explain their responses to the system. The medical record folder will typically include the following elements:

1. Letters from the referring GP and/or consultant.

2. Patient data entered by the nurses (i.e. height, weight, blood pressure, etc.).

3. The hand-written case notes relating to any previous outpatient visits.

4. The laboratory results (e.g. biochemistry, haematology).

5. Copies of the letters sent to the GPs (or referring consultants) concerning the patient ('clinic letter').

In addition, the medical records on patients who had previously been an inpatient, would include the additional material:

6. The case notes relating to the inpatient stay(s), include a full 'clerking'.

7. The operation notes in the case of patients who had undergone surgical procedures.

8. A copy of the discharge summary which includes the final diagnosis.

9. Any referral letters to members of any 'other disciplines' involved with the care of the patient (e.g. social workers, physiotherapists).

These documents were kept in a standard numbered medical record folder and filed in the medical records office when not in use.

Turning to the COSTAR system itself, the programmes were supplied from the USA free of charge while the hardware and technical support were made available by the Regional Health Authority (RHA) at very little cost. This inexpensiveness was a consequence of the American developers being keen to promote it and the RHA having adopted the MUMPS programming language on which it was based as standard software for clinical system.

The system replaced the hand-written case notes by a printed form, known as the encounter form. These forms consisted of pre-coded lists of signs, symptoms, diagnoses, operations, investigations and drugs as well as space for narrative information (Figure 5.5). The doctors where intended to complete the encounter form at the time of seeing the patient in the clinic (medical encounter). At the end of the clinic the completed forms would be collected by the nurses and passed to one of the data-entry clerks and the data could then be input onto the system. Prior to the next clinic an encounter report (Figure 5.6) consisting of summaries of the patients' case notes and investigations would be printed and inserted into the medical record folder.

The new (COSTAR) system presented patient information in a format that was much more systematic and comprehensive than was previously the case. At the same time the system demanded the doctors changed the way they recorded and recalled patient information and data in the clinic. It was the effects these changes of the clinical information systems had on medical work that caused the doctors ultimately to reject the system. It was also the case that some consultants concluded that the alliance they had formed with Dr Old was not helping them to achieve their own objectives. A situation readily analyzable in terms of Latour's (1987) actor network model. The coalition of doctors could not hold because it proved impossible to integrate the interests of them all (*intéressement*) to ensure their sufficient commitment (*enrolment*) to guarantee none would renege on their agreement (*mobilization*). Even so the collegiality of the consultants ensured that their rejection of the system would not be interpreted as a failure but as a

PRESENTING COMPLAINT AND OTHER MAJOR SYMPTOMS					
	ALIMENTARY SYSTEM				
1 2 3	Abdo. pain Appetite poor Diarrhoea	PHBFI DHBT2 PDKV1	12 13 14	Angina Chest pain Haemoptysis	NMBK4 NHBV1 MHDY6
DIAGNOSIS					
	ALIMENTARY SYSTEM			ENDO/ METABOLIC	
41 42 43	Crohns Colitis Cirrhosis	PKIQ1-1 PKIZ1-A PMK1	64 65 66	Diabetes Hyperthyroid Hyperlipidaemia	FIBT2 EGLD6 FINS3
COMMENTS					
OTHER SYSTEMS					
ALLERGIES					
SOCIAL HISTORY					
PHYSICAL EXAMINATION Appearance/facies/skin/hair/thyroid					DCBN1
Lymph nodes/Swelling					DCMS1
Mouth, pharynx, ears					DCBO1
	INVESTIGATIONS			**DRUGS**	
 4 5	BIOCHEMISTRY Cardiac enzymes Creatinine	 DOEY5 DOEQ5	 36 37	 Tetracycline Thyroxine	 ETFL1 FUDA1

Figure 5.5 Extract from a COSTAR encounter form - general medicine

(*Note: The alpha-numeric codes are fictitious*)

```
ENCOUNTER REPORT UN: 123456N        PRINTED 4/1/89
SMITH, SHEILA(F) 73YRS (7/2/22)

25/11/81 SITE: ST GILES             TYPE:SCHED.VISIT
         FIRST ATTEND.GP REFERRAL   OLD, P. DR

                DISPOSITIONS

BBDR1    DISPOSITION  APPOINTMENT IN 1 WEEKS TIME
                                        WITH DR OLD

              DIAGNOSIS/PROBLEMS
NIBC1    HYPERTENSION [MAJOR]
YHGO4-1  JOINT PAIN
            PAIN INNER LEFT THIGH, INTERMITTENT
            EXCRUCIATING PAINS ESP WALKING
DHBE1    DEBILITY [MAJOR]
            MULTIPLE COMPLAINTS, TEETH, WHITLOW,
            PAIN EVERYWHERE, NAUSEA ETC. 'FEELS
            THAT LIFE'S A DRAG'.
CMTC1    SYSTEMS REVIEW
            CVS - OCCASIONAL CHEST PAINS = PILLS-
            FOOD, RT ANKLE SWELLING. RESP.- BREATH-
            LESS ... INDIGESTION ... APPETITE FAIR.
            WEIGHT > BOWELS CONSTIPATED, GU -
            ACHING LOWER ABDO. ... SLEEPS WELL ...
DNRM1    PAST MEDICAL HISTORY ALLERGIES
            HYPERTENSION DIAGNOSED 1984,
            HYSTERECTOMY @ 37YRS ST GILES ...
            CARPLE TUNNEL SYNDROME RELEASE X 2
            BILAT, MANIP. OF L.HIP ST PETER'S
            HOSPITAL
CMHS1    FAMILY HISTORY
            OLDER BROTHER WELL. FATHER DIED HEART
            TROUBLE, MOTHER DIED PA.
```

Figure 5.6 Extract from a fictional COSTAR encounter report (continued next page)

(This extract is for illustrative purposes only. All details are fictitious)

```
CMTK2    SOCIAL HISTORY - SMOKING NIL.ALCOHOL NIL.
            JOB HOUSEWIFE
CMEG1    DRUGS
            PIROXICAM 10MG BD. NORMAX. ISOGEL.
            LORAZEPAM 1MG TDS. BELLERGAL ...
            ? DOSE 2. NITRAZEPAM 5MG NOCTE.
DCBN1    APPEARANCE FACIES SKIN HAIR THYROID
            LOOKS DEPRESSED/ASLEEP
VKZL1    ANXIETY [MAJOR]
CMCD2    NO CODE 1 - IATROGENIC - TOO MANY PILLS

                 PHYSICAL EXAM
DBKD1    HEIGHT                      167
DBLI1    WEIGHT                      79.4
DBEB1    PULSE                       80
DBFGI *  BLOOD PRESSURE              150/100
DCMS1    LYMPH NODES SWELLINGS
            NONE BUT PAINFUL SWELLING MEDIAL
            ASPECT  LEFT THIGH SEE DIAG. IN NOTES
DCIB1    HANDS NAILS                 NAD
RCBO1    MOUTH PHARYNX EARS          NAD
MCMK1    LUNGS

                   THERAPIES
SSKN4    MODURETIC - 2 TABLETS MANE
OYCO6     DIET - WT REDUCING

                     TESTS
DMBS7    BLOOD UREA                  5.5
DMCF1    SERUM SODIUM                134
DMCK2    SERUM POTASSIUM (ETC)       ...
DMGB1 *  SERUM CALCIUM (ETC)         2.16

         ADMINISTRATIVE
BSED2-M  MARITAL STATUS              MARRIED
BTBQ2    PATIENT'S OCCUPATION        HOUSEWIFE
```

Figure 5.6 Extract from a fictional COSTAR encounter report (continued)

(*This extract is for illustrative purposes only. All details are fictitious*) particular variety of 'rhetorical closure' (Pinch and Bijker, 1984; 1987). How this came about is my next concern.

Each consultant was invited by Dr Old to design their own encounter forms with his help. In the event the more committed consultant from each of the specialties carried out this work on behalf of her or his colleagues. The consultants were brought on to the system singly and in pairs over a period of twelve months. The system was further developed and modified during the implementation period largely as a result of comments and criticisms of the consultants.

The consultants responses to using the system, changed over time. At the outset all the consultants supported the proposal. By July, 1982, however, all the consultants (excepting Dr Old) had decided not to continue with the system. The responses of the junior medical staff were similar. The consultants' commitment was based primarily on their sense of professional collegiality but the strength of this support varied greatly in terms of whether they believed the system could be instrumental in furthering their own schemes. There is, however, an important distinction to be made between the politics of (collegiate) commitment (*intéressement*) and the pragmatism of recording case notes. It was when the consultants' realised that their clinic routines were prejudiced by the new computer system they began to withdraw their active support.

The doctors' responses (both consultants and junior staff) broadly followed a trajectory of initial *acceptance* leading to a degree of *compliance* in completing the encounter forms. Then, following some experience with the system of data capture and its reports, some junior doctors sought ways of *resisting* the system's requirements while the consultants gradually moved to a position of *rejecting* the system. But, interestingly, they did so in such a way that it did not appear to be unsupportive of their colleague, Dr Old', or his computer project. There was, however, considerable variation between the consultants in terms of the pace at which they moved through the stages. The trajectory of responses to the COSTAR system will now be discussed in a little more detail in order that the reasons for the variation between consultants and between consultants and junior medical staff can be better understood.

Acceptance Collegiality was a major factor influencing the co-operation of the consultants. This was so to such a degree that some would struggle to complete the encounter forms even though their design was completely at variance with their own practice. The cause of the problem was not the computer system as such but originated in the encounter form having been designed by the colleague in the same specialty and who adopted a very different approach to case notes. In the case of urology, for instance, the one who designed the form wrote very brief technical notes focusing solely on the patient's malfunctioning urological system while the other took the more holistic view that 'there is an awful lot that is not urological that comes into the history-taking'. Even after using the system for over a year s/he still found that, '... it ... makes everything that much ..longer and (more) complicated'.

Compliance The junior doctors were not consulted over the introduction of COSTAR they were simply expected to comply with its requirements. In consequence, it would be more accurate to define these doctors' acceptance of the system as compliance. Nearly half of all the junior doctors interviewed (Total: 22) were able to identify some benefits from the system's introduction. In general these were seen as compensations for having to use the system. The general opinion, however, was summed up by the comment 'when the present system works perfectly well its hard to see benefits ...'.

Resistance Despite the general lack of commitment only one junior doctor ever openly resisted its use. S/he would 'clerk' new patients in the traditional narrative format on the encounter form completely ignoring the listing of coded signs, symptoms (etc.). The matter was brought to the attention of Dr Old by one of the computer clerks who spoke with the consultant who then admonished the junior doctor. Other junior doctors learnt from this episode and would take paper with them to clinic so as to covertly 'clerk' patients in the traditional format prior to transferring the information to the encounter form. The rationale for this practice was twofold. Firstly, these doctors felt more in control 'clerking' rather than filling in a form. Secondly, the technique was of far greater use to them in the longer term. COSTAR was specific to this hospital's outpatient department whereas traditional 'clerking' was a universal practice.

Rejection One consultant did refuse to use the system from the very beginning but even s/he officially supported the proposal for reasons of collegiate solidarity. This consultant, a rheumatologist, had a manual system that contained over a decade's worth of data on drugs and laboratory tests as well as a unique clinical scoring system for assessing a patient's condition. S/he was not prepared to risk the integrity of this system by taking on the additional burden of using COSTAR. The odd thing about this matter was that the manual card system was based on numerically data and technically which technically could have easily been computerized. This was not possible organizationally, however, because the COSTAR project lacked the resources necessary to include the clinical research activities of individual consultants and especially not 10 years of data. In important part the fate of the COSTAR system was tied to the inability of Dr Old to provide additional facilities desired by the consultants. What several really wanted was for the system to provide support for their various clinical research projects. At least four of the consultants maintained separate (dual) records, in addition to that kept in the medical record folder, for clinical, research and audit purposes. In addition to the rheumatology data-base, already mentioned, there were card systems for urology, surgical audit and one for a subset of gynaecological patients. Excepting the rheumatologist these consultants were the strongest supporters of the COSTAR system who designed the encounter forms for their specialties. These consultants were the instrumentally committed ones who had anticipated that their card systems would be transferred onto COSTAR. When it became obvious that this was not going to happen they withdraw from the project although in a manner that made it appear that the rejection was only a modification to the system of data capture ('closure by redefinition').

The other and not unrelated reason for the rejection of COSTAR was on the grounds that it demanded too radical a change in the way that doctors wrote and used case notes. As one consultant explained:

> It gradually dawned on me ... [in] clinic after clinic I have to 'skip' the [printed] 'status reports' and [laboratory] results and go to the [original] investigation form ... and ... my letter to the GP [i.e. 'clinic letter']. And I really miss *writing outpatient notes in my own handwriting [and] looking at this in my next clinic*, this to me conveys continuity, somehow sheet after sheet of computer data means nothing when it comes to clinical work. (*emphases added*)

This emphasis on the writing and subsequent reading of case notes within the medical encounter as an integral part of the clinic process was also reported by the other consultants. One argued that the COSTAR system interfered with the 'thought process in clinical diagnosis ... the system of recording the database [on the encounter form] seem[ed] to act as a wedge'. Actually, this consultant relied on an SHO to act as an amanuensis to complete the Encounter forms and correct them after the clinic. Nevertheless, other consultants also found it inconvenient because of the mismatch between what the system was designed to do and what the consultants thought they wanted it to do.

The final rejection of the system, however, was more real than apparent. It was formally agreed by the Hospital Medical Committee that the Encounter forms would be replaced by the traditional case notes which the computer clerks would encode prior to entry onto the computer data-base. The minute read as follows:

> [C]ertain consultants did not necessarily wish to continue using the system as originally designed. ... [although] it was quite apparent that support for the system still existed ... [I]t was agreed that the future use of the Encounter form would be reviewed and if possible a system designed that was perhaps less invasive in terms of the preparation of patients notes.

This encapsulates the ambiguity of the consultants towards the project. On the one hand, they have no wish to undermine a colleagues research (*collegiate solidarity*), while on the other, they have no desire to continue with the COSTAR system if it was not going to provide them with additional facilities. Hence the compromise. They even agreed to accept some of the printed reports although neither the consultants nor the junior staff used (excepting occasions when the medical record was missing). To quote one consultant gynaecologist, '[there] is now ... a blank sheet and I just write ... what I want recorded ... I [do] have investigations [printed] at the back [but] drugs I just put down at the end of my blank sheet - that is perfectly satisfactory. *What I do not like ... is the printout*' (*emphases in original*). Thus the COSTAR system was formally found to be acceptable to the doctors although in reality they had been rejected it. It was a case of 'closure by redefinition' brought about by the instability of the (medical) actor network.

The structure and process of writing case notes

Long before the introduction of COSTAR at St Giles Bittner and Garfinkel (1967, p.206) had demonstrated the cryptic nature of clinic records. Moreover, they also pointed out that such records can only be 'read' with the 'insider knowledge' of the particular clinic. According to these authors the underlying reason for this was that of economy i.e. whether the collection of the information was worth the effort (ibid., pp.192-4). Selection of data was determined by what was considered minimally necessary in order for the doctors' to function effectively (ibid., p.194). The politics of information control ('keeping the front office appropriately misinformed') was seen as only a subordinate reason (ibid., p.194). The authors argued that clinic records might be read either as a record of a 'therapeutic contract' or as an 'actuarial record' even though the two readings were irreconcilable (ibid., p.198).

The capacity for the records to deliver accurate data for actuarial purposes (i.e. aggregate analysis for management or research purposes) was very limited because it was the 'therapeutic contract' (i.e. medico-legal purposes) that took precedence (ibid., p.199). They argued that it was out of the fragments of information, in combination with a knowledge of the organization of the clinic, that a clinician could reconstitute the information required whether for clinical or legal reasons (ibid., pp.202-5). The technique, it was argued, was the same as for a lawyer when s/he, 'makes a brief' (ibid., p.203). This approach should not, be read as being a case intentional misrepresentation for it is not 'governed by personal considerations in advancing a cause' (ibid., p.200). The account clearly referred to normal everyday arrangements and was not an exposé of bad practice.

The doctors at St Giles Hospital shared at least some of the suppositions of their American colleagues studied by Bittner and Garfinkel. The consultants tended to be neither comprehensive nor routinely systematic in writing case notes. The clinical information was only rendered into a systematic record when, typically, the 'clinic letter' was written. This arrangement was overlooked by the consultants when they designed the encounter forms. The encounter forms were designed to capture most eventualities in a way that was easiest to input onto the data-base and not with the doctors' own method of working. As one consultant remarked, 'I still find it rather bewildering particularly when I am ... looking around for where the symptoms are [on the form] ... I feel very much like a Chinese waiter'.

In general doctors are taught to write case notes in the following way. First the doctor will record details of the patient's history (basically the 'presenting complaint' of the patient, past medical history, social history, drug history) and physical examination. At which stage s/he will decide on an initial ('presumptive') diagnosis, or some other equivalent assessment of the patient's condition. On the basis of this the doctor will order any laboratory or clinical investigations believed necessary, recommend medically appropriate therapy and, in the case of an outpatients' clinic, write a letter to the patient's general practitioner or other referring doctor (the 'clinic letter'). Patients returning for further visits ('follow up' patients) would typically warrant only brief entries in the case notes concerning any changes in the patient's condition or treatment.

There were, however, considerable variations between consultants and specialties with many case notes apparently incomplete or indecipherable. There was also a significant difference between the methods of the consultants and those of the junior doctors. This was not a situation peculiar to the St Giles outpatients' department. In the Bittner and Garfinkel study (1967) the authors identified the overriding priority as being medico-legal. This interpretation, however, did not explain the situation at St Giles Hospital. The major reasons for the cryptic nature of case notes were not related to medical defensiveness but, as it turned out, time economy and pragmatism. Overall it was possible to identify four rationales that informed the doctors use of case notes within the clinics:

1. medico-legal;
2. education and research;
3. training and monitoring;
4. decision aid.

Each will be explained in turn.

Case notes as medico-legal documents Medical records (including the case notes) are legally owned by the Secretary of State and are not the property of the doctors who makes the record (Home Office, 1978, para. 7.11). When the case notes are signed by a doctor they have a legal status and constitute evidence of medical work carried out or planned for the future. Yet only one of the consultants took the legal status into account when writing in the case notes. S/he would record criticisms of other doctors to, 'protect myself from litigation because someone has given absolutely the wrong treatment'. One other consultant did point out 'that something may happen [to a patient] and ultimately end in the coroners court ... Then [the clinic record] needs to look reasonably clear'. No other consultant, however, expressed concern concerning the possibility of litigation and it played little part in the way the consultants or the junior medical staff wrote their case notes.

Case notes for educational and research purposes In order for the case notes to be of use as a research resource they would need to be recorded systematically and comprehensively. Some hospitals are renowned for the completeness and consistency of their medical records. One famous example is the Massachusetts General Hospital in the USA which has maintained detailed records since 1821 (Reiser, 1978, pp.206-8). On this side of the Atlantic no hospital has earned a similar reputation, although certain specialties within specific hospitals have implemented at different times a policy of comprehensive, detailed records as, for example, in the case of Surgery at Guy's Hospital in the 1970s (McColl et al., 1976, p.1342). There was no such policy at St Giles. Nevertheless, there was a practical need for the clinic records to be maintained as a research resource. Registrars were expected (as part of their training) to carry out research which would involve them searching through the case notes of selected patient groups. The registrars did not anticipate that the records would be complete or reliable. Instead they relied more on any systematically recorded numerical data contained within the medical record (e.g. laboratory results) although even this data could be unreliable because it was often misplaced or lost. Preparation for case-meetings would also cause the registrars to turn to the case notes for research-type information. Registrars in the surgical specialties were expected to regularly present cases at the weekly meetings. The objective of these meetings was primarily educational 'essentially it is one of student teaching, interesting and abnormal cases [which can be] shown well on X-rays ...' (Consultant). This would not entail the routine writing of systematic and comprehensive case notes. 'Interesting' cases invariably involved an inpatient stay and with it the opportunity for a comprehensive 'clerking' and a full set of investigations.

Consultants with an interest in research or audit would ensure that the relevant data was recorded on documents other than the case notes, as one explained to me '... I have .. a diagnostic index cabinet in which I put all letters and patient records - not the patient record- my own copies ... I [can] go and ... pick-up "gallstones" [for example] in the last ten years'. This practice of maintaining dual systems was not an uncommon one.

Case notes for training and monitoring junior medical staff On the wards house officers are responsible for 'clerking' the new patients. Much of these doctor's training centres on learning how to conduct a history and examination making a ('presumptive') diagnosis (Rees, 1981, pp.56-9). In outpatients' clinics this training element is not routinely present. If house staff were to fully 'clerk' all new patients it would greatly reduce the number of patients seen. At St Giles there were two consultants who included a training element in the house officers clinic work. The first was the general physician who arranged the clinics such that the SHOs 'clerked' all the new patients. Second was one of the gynaecologists who used the outpatients' clinics as settings in which to train medical students in the art of case note writing. There was also the urologist who wrote all the clinic letters 'and check what [the junior doctors] have said ...'. in order to 'control[..] what goes on between the GPs and the junior staff.' It was a method unique to this consultant.

Case notes as a decision aid The main rationale for writing case notes was as part of the clinical decision-making process. The degree of detail a doctor would include would vary according to, firstly, the nature of the problem and, secondly, the seniority and experience of the doctor. A registrar for example, explained that, ' ... if [a patient] comes in with a lump under their arm, you write down "cyst" and that is probably the end of it, but if it is more serious then a more comprehensive record is made'. Even so, no registrar would, '... write such detailed notes at 'outpatients' as a house [officer] would when they are admitting a patient. [Instead they would] only ask questions relevant to the particular problem'. It was, however, the usual method of the house staff '...[to] go through every ... system in the body' when dealing with new patients. This helped ensure the doctor would not overlook anything of significance and had the added advantage of simultaneously underpinning his or her social ascendancy within the encounter simply by setting the agenda for the interaction (e.g. Waitzkin and Stoeckle, 1976, p.265). Registrarship was, according to those interviewed, the stage at which doctors began to move away from the comprehensiveness of 'clerking' and towards the idiosyncratic brevity characteristic of many of the consultants.

The consultants never took full patient histories but instead focused principally on the patient's 'presenting complaint'. It was this that formed the organizing principle to their note-taking. There were, however, important differences between the methods adopted by physicians and surgeons. As one consultant explained:

> Physicians ... are likely to do 'notes' in outpatients more on the ... systematic format of the archetypal 'clerking' of a patient ... [T]he majority of surgical clinics ... are too big to devote much time to each patient ... I go straight into the main complaint then take any relevant ... history.

The point about the physicians was only partially accurate, for as one explained: 'I make notes which are meaningful to me ... I tend to have a statement to begin [on] how a person looks ... then I go for the particular things that are important... To get to the guts of the case quickly ...' Generally, the consultants wrote brief observations to assist them arrive at a conclusion as how best they would manage the patient. These notes then formed the basis (an *aide memoire*) for the 'clinic letter' dictated after the clinic. As one consultant commented, 'trying to get information out of the body of 'notes' which is in somebody else's writing - and someone else's paragraphing - is extremely difficult ... '. One of the gynaecologists explained, 'outpatients' clinics are notoriously dangerous places for missing out information any patient being admitted has to be reassessed on admission ... to make sure we are doing the right thing'.

Nevertheless, the doctors had developed strategies for eliciting reasonably useful information from the case notes. The main technique used by junior doctors and consultants alike were to refer directly to the clinic letter. While the 'clinic letter' was usually the first point of reference it was not, however, the only document referred to. Doctors might also refer to a range of other documentation contained within the medical records including, for example, in the case of surgery, 'investigation results, discharge summaries, operation notes and the inpatient notes'. Most consultants had developed their own techniques of speeding up this procedure, typically by 'the actual paragraphing ...' (Rheumatologist), 'notations and underlining important points' (Urologist).

In contradistinction to Bittner and Garfinkel's analysis the COSTAR case study indicates that medical records, at least in the British context, implicitly possess not two but four medical rationales and it is the decision aid rationale that is the paramount one. In practice this has little to do with the technical details of medical decision-making and more with what Bloor (1976b, p.45) has called:

> [T]hose idiosyncratically developed rules of thumb concerning those particular symptoms and signs which the specialist feels to be typically minimally acceptable criterion for allocating [patients] to the various alternative forms of therapeutic intervention at his disposal.

These rules are constructed with the intention of avoiding what Scheff (1978, p.609) has termed a Type 1 error ('to dismiss a patient who is actually ill'). Unlike 'clerking', neither the criteria for the use of medical evidence nor the line of reasoning adopted are other than the doctor's own (based on medical knowledge and clinical experience). This means that the experienced doctor is freed from the need to follow a rigid format of history-taking, examination and investigations but can approach those facets of the medical encounter with considerable flexibility to save time and reinforce the patient's confidence in the chosen course of treatment. The use of the medical record in this way facilitates and represents an aspect of 'face-work' (Goffman, 1972; Strong, 1979, p.40) and is an integral part of the process of maintaining the doctor's autonomy.

The general argument here is commensurate with Bloor's (1976b, p.45) use of the term decision rules. The evidence from the case study indicates that it is the actual process of writing the case notes that typically aids the doctor in deciding on which of 'the various alternative forms of therapeutic intervention [to adopt]' (ibid.). The notes are meant for posterity but to assist in assessing whether the 'minimally acceptable criterion' (ibid.) had been reached, or not. They are also the tangible expression of the consultant's autonomy and are, in a strict sense, only accessible to her/his interpretation. This selective approach gives the consultant, in particular, great flexibility within the medical encounter. It can be used either save time in a busy clinic, or reinforce the patient's confidence in the doctor and hospital (by the doctor concentrating on the patient's own perception of his or her complaint). One of the physicians at St Giles, for example, would include in her case notes, 'other things that are domestically relevant that patients [mention] ... so that next time you can say "you went to Blackpool last year" and the patient suddenly thinks you're wonderful ... and any treatment you give is more likely to work'. Unlike 'clerking' proper the line of reasoning is pragmatic and not predetermined. Whatever form the case notes take the consultant remains the arbiter of her or his own medical performance. If a doctor wants to find out what a colleague had decided regarding a particular patient it is not to the case notes he or she would first refer, but to the 'clinic letter'.

It was because of the incompatibility between these well-established methods of writing and accessing case notes by doctors' and that programmed by the COSTAR system that the computer system failed. It was of little use to the doctors as a decision aid nor could it be relied upon to underpin their autonomy and therefore their ascendancy within the medical encounter.

Much has changed within the NHS since the completion of the case study and particularly relevant here has been the increasing government pressure on doctors to be more accountable for their clinical work. A central issue here has been the one of medical audit which would appear to require systematic and complete clinic notes (as evidence of good practice). This, in turn, would make the records more accessible to automation. Yet the way that medical audit has been introduced does not suggest that doctors have found it necessary, at least not yet, to change their record keeping procedures. It is this topic of medical audit I now turn.

Medical computing and professional autonomy II: The case of medical audit and the new management systems

The introduction of the 'internal market' within the NHS has meant that the issue of quality control has come to occupy centre stage in relations between purchasers and providers. Purchasers want evidence that the quality of care is commensurate to its cost. This is an issue that directly impinges on clinical work as medical audit. This and related terms will be clarified in the next sub-section. The general purpose of this part of the chapter is to explore in some detail the issue of medical audit and only then the role played by IT. For without an awareness of the occupational and organizational politics of medical audit the limited IT support and general lack of integration with wider information systems make little sense.

Medical audit, quality assurance and clinical autonomy

The UK medical profession only recently embraced medical audit despite the issue having been around for a considerable time. It has done so only after firm direction from government in the 1989 'White Paper' (HMSO, 1989a and b) and subsequent *NHS and Community Care Act*, 1990 plus the input of a reasonably substantial amount money from the Department of Health: £28 million in 1989/91, £48 million in 1991/92 and £42 million in 1992/93 a total of £118 million (Department of Health, 1993). This funding being principally required to cover the salaries of audit support staff and IT equipment (Packwood et al., 1994, p.308).

Yet medical audit is no recent innovation. It has been a *leitmotiv* of profession/state relations since the 1960s (Dent, 1995a) and in its modern form, is premised on a systems model developed in the USA initially by Donabedian (1966). The model comprises of three elements, *structure, process* and *outcome* that together define the components of medical audit within modern medicine. In addition, there should also be a 'feedback loop' from *outcome* to *structure* in order to ensure that lessons learnt from the activity of audit do lead to changes in the organization and delivery of medical care (see Figure 5.7).

The medical profession has generally preferred medical audit of the 'process' kind as it can remain directly under their control for only they can be the judge of a doctor's performance (Donabedian, 1966, p.168; Shaw, 1980a). It is also the case that it can be exceedingly difficult to derive feasible measures of outcome (Butler and Vaile, 1984, pp.127-8) because it is often difficult to (a) identify the precise outcome sought (e.g. extend life or improve its quality), (b) establish the causal links between treatment and outcome and (c) acquire the data once patients have left hospital. Yet this is precisely the area which current medical audit practices are intended to address (Orchard, 1994, p.1493).

Traditionally, British doctors have tended to treat medical audit with great circumspection (Dent, 1995). Its modern origins stem from the National Standardization Programme for hospitals back in 1919 which was set in train by the American College of Surgeons (ACS)· Originally they were littlc more than 'case meetings' or 'chart reviews'. The surgical specialities in the US and UK subsequently developed the routine practice of holding morbidity and mortality meetings that reviewed work of each 'firm'. Some observers have argued that these events function less as an audit than as a means of socializing neophyte doctors (Bosk, 1979) and provide an opportunity for catharsis for those doctors unfortunate enough to have a patient die whilst under their care (Arluke, 1977; Millman, 1977). In other words, the meetings function more to strengthen professional autonomy than as a clinical accounting exercise.

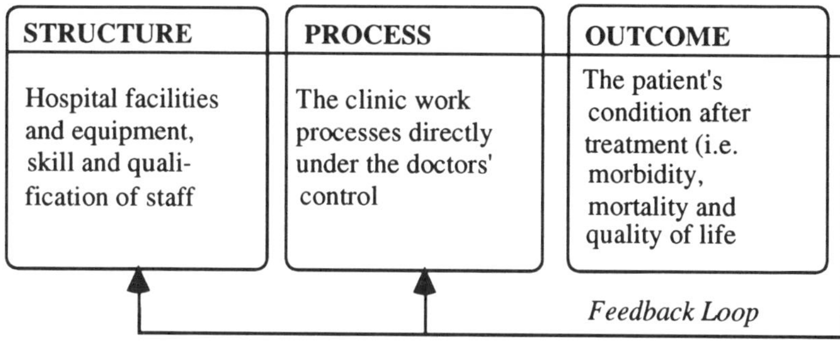

Figure 5.7 The medical audit model

(Based on Donabedian, 1966)

Physicians, by contrast, have limited their own involvement in the assessment of the quality of medical care (as distinct to medical audit) to case reviews. These have been primarily used for educational and training purposes and the presentation of medically 'interesting' cases rather than for audit purposes. Change began to be put in train in the US in the mid 1960s. The pressure for medical audit in all specialties (medical as well as surgical) came as the result of upwardly spiralling health costs that followed the introduction of the Medicare and Medicaid programmes in 1965. The initial response was the introduction of utilization reviews. These were designed to be checks on the cost efficiency of the treatments given. The system, however, proved to be too cumbersome and expensive (Freidson, 1976; McSherry, 1976). This ultimately led to a change of emphasis from costs to the quality of care (Dent, 1995). The new system of evaluation was based on explicit, written, criteria (or protocols) which are established beforehand (by the senior medical staff) and 'policed' by the medical audit committee within the hospital (Sanazaro, 1974, p.272; Shaw, 1980b, p.1510). In the US it is the medical records staff who monitor the clinic records for the medical audit committee. In practice, at least in the early days of the new system, the issue of incomplete records was a major problem (Sanazaro, 1974, p.272).

This change of emphasis from cost to quality was the result, at least in part, of the American Medical Association's (AMA) strategy to avoid outside controls being applied to the profession (Westin, 1976, p.54; Krause, 1977, pp.290-3). Nevertheless, the implementation of the federally mandated peer review met with considerable hostility from the membership (Björkman, 1989, p.55). A similar situation subsequently emerged in Britain (Dent, 1993).

In the UK national audit systems have existed for some time for certain specific patient groups. A very good illustration of this is the national

Confidential Enquiry into Maternal Deaths (Godber, 1976; Butler and Vaile, 1984, pp.168-9) which has been in existence since 1952. There is now also the more recent Confidential Enquiry into Perioperative Deaths (CEPOD), which is much cited as 'good practice' (e.g. HMSO, 1989b, p.4). Another initiative is the Oxford Medical Record Linkage system which is a computer-based system that inter-links the medical records at different hospitals in order to provide a comprehensive patient data-base (Henderson *et al.,* 1989).

These examples, however, are the exceptions. Doctors in the UK have generally and consistently been adverse to the introduction of medical audit even when their own professional association advocated it as a means of resisting state encroachment (Dent, 1995). Even so the British Medical Association (BMA) equivocated over the issue of medical audit in its evidence to the 1979 Royal Commission (Merrison, 1979), commenting that 'its place ... in health care is still controversial' but if it was to be inevitable it should be carried out by the profession as a whole (BMJ Supplement, 1977, p.301). The BMA also regretted 'any suggestion that there should be "medical audit" by the state' (ibid.). The Royal Commission was not impressed and in the report commented, '... we are not convinced that the profession generally regards the introduction of audit or peer review ... with a proper sense of urgency' (Merrison, 1979, para. 12.56). It recommended that, 'a planned programme for the introduction of audit or peer review ... should be set up for the health professions by their professional bodies and progress monitored by the health departments' (ibid., para.63). This was exactly what was contained in the 'White Paper' (HMSO, 1989a) and Working Paper 6 (HMSO, 1989b).

At about the time of the 'White Paper' studies reported by Harrison and Schulz (1989, p.203) revealed that British doctors 'regard overall financial limitations as being legitimate restrictions on their autonomy ... [but] did not see a legitimate role for ... peer review or quality assurance'. Under the requirements of the 'White Paper', however, 'audit' was an essential requirement although a distinction was made between medical and clinical types of audit. The former related only to the work of the clinicians while the latter concerned the whole health care team (Shaw and Costain, 1989; DoH, 1994). Whilst medical audit systems were implemented at hospital level by 1993 the NHS Management Executive had decided to switch the emphasis and its funding from medical audit to clinical audit (NHS. ME., 1993) a policy which comes into effect in 1995/96 (NHS. ME., 1994). An important consideration for the NHS Management Executive was that this broader based approach would enable the audit to 'be informed by purchaser/provider and public/patient as well as professional (college) priorities' (NHS ME., 1993 Appendix B 'Principles and Vision'). In other words, the strategy is one of trying to ensure that quality of medical work does come under routine management scrutiny (along with the work of other hospital professionals) which did not seem to be happening with any speed under the medical audit model. Similarly, the intention is to 'ensure that the information and IT needs of audit are integrated into wider unit [e.g. hospital] based information and IT strategies (including resource management and HISS)' (NHS ME., 1993, Annex B, p.2) which is not the case under the medical audit arrangements as has been clearly demonstrated by Kerrison et al (1993) in their recent study.

Since the publication of 'Working Paper 6 (HMSO, 1989b, para. 2.3) 'outcome' measures have become the central issue and it would seem that the difficulties outlined earlier are no longer considered insurmountable by the policy advisers. Already work has being published on the use of 're-admission rates' as just such an indicator and one that is relatively uncomplicated to measure (Henderson et al., 1989, pp.709-13; Greener, 1989, pp.12-13). There is also some evidence that work is being carried out to introduce GP reporting systems where patients are treated at the GP clinic for infections and the like following hospital treatment (e.g. DoH, 1994, p.25). These approaches may be useful for acute cases but in the area of chronic illness 'outcome' is less certain and more a matter of the alleviation of suffering than the curing of the disease. Moreover, the 're-admission rates' approach fails to identify patients' qualitative dissatisfactions with the outcome which would, in any case be difficult to measure (Cochrane, 1971; Illsley, 1980; Butler and Vaile, 1984). Nevertheless, the Royal Colleges now view 'outcome' as the most relevant indicator for medical audit purposes (e.g. Royal College of Physicians, 1989, para. 2.4). Despite this formal commitment of the Royal Colleges to outcome measures, however, much emphasis remains on process audit as Shaw and Costain (1989, p.498) indicate in a passage that neatly distinguishes audit from related clinical activities:

> [M]edical audit relates to practices initiated directly by doctors. It ... is primarily clinical ... its focus is the *process and results* of medical care ... Medical audit is more systematic, quantified, and formal than traditional clinical ward rounds, meetings, and case presentations but shares with these the objectives of better patient care and education (*Emphases added*)

Moreover, to be 'systematic [and] quantified' routine medical care has to be regularly 'logged' within the medical records but, as has been demonstrated earlier, this does not happen although changes are being made to meet the new requirements. Hospitals and specialties are beginning to include audit forms in the medical records folders so that data may be routinely collected (Interviews, 1995) but this does not appear to be the general case and there is generally a 'lack of routinely collected ... data for the purpose of monitoring quality' (Kerrison, 1993, p.150). Instead, the system is seen as being limited in scope, not integrated into patterns of work and isolated from other management and quality assurance activities (Kerrison, et al., 1993, p.1). The sentence just cited actually refers to 'computerized data' (Kerrison, 1993, p.150). Only 10 per cent of the medical audit support staff included in the Brunel study (Kerrison et al., 1993, p.51) reported using a case-mix management system and 20 per cent an order communication system in an audit. On the other hand, 70 per cent of the medical audit staff routinely retrieved data from case notes (ibid., p.58, Table 10). According to the report (ibid., p.59):

> The issue of information technology is ... vexed ... some staff identified the lack of their own information technology which made audit time consuming ... [T]his lack also meant that access to information and to computers for processing information had to be negotiated with other departments. These may be unsympathetic or have other priorities.

The recent Audit Commission report on information management (1995a) reported further evidence of a similar kind. One of the hospital trusts visited had forty separate audit systems that did not interlink with any other. This apparent extreme IT isolationism needs to be considered along with Kerrison's (1993) finding that on occasions, 'preoccupation with information technology ... detracted from undertaking "proper" audits. Comments ... included: ".. *consultants cannot grasp the philosophy of standard-setting if there is a computer around*"' (ibid., p.59, *emphases in original*). Yet the alternative strategy of reliance on manual case notes seriously restricts the collection of large data-sets needed for effectively auditing. Medical audit has been more successful in its medical education and training role providing 'a forum for members of a common profession, motivated by a common desire to provide appropriate medicine '(ibid., p.45). By the same token this may well be one of the reasons for the NHS Management Executive switching its emphasis from medical to clinical audit (NHS. ME., 1993 and 1994). Nevertheless, whether medical audit is a formal, systematic and quantified monitoring system or an improved system of education and training '[r]eviewing quality and taking corrective action ... helps reduce costs' (Enthoven, 1985, p.44). It is, therefore, hardly surprising that the government was to use the National Audit Office and the Public Accounts Committee as the means of assessing the general quality of care within the NHS (NAO, 1988; PAC, 1989). The NAO was concerned from the outset to investigate the issue of medical audit in relation to the financial management of the NHS (1988, p.1, para. 1) while the PAC concluded that it might be necessary for audit to be covered through some form of contractual arrangement (1989, p.vii, para. 9). District health authorities, in assessing which hospitals to contract with, would then have to take the quality of care - as well as price - into account. The evidence from the Brunel study was that this has not yet occurred and that medical audit has remained primarily a system of peer review and professional socialization. The more recent decisions reflected in the NHS Management Executive's circulars (1993 and 1994) indicates that the policy emphasis will be to switch the audit focus from the medical model to the multi-disciplinary clinical one and thereby avoid the potential for conflict between doctors and managers and in the process establish a means of integrating the activities of all professional groups involved in hospital care including the nurses and the professions allied to medicine.

Conclusions

The evidence presented in this chapter all points to doctors retaining their autonomy in face of any rationalizing tendencies associated with the introduction or extension of clinical and hospital systems. Generally doctors have favoured those computer systems used to support research activities or education and training. New computer systems, however, have proven to be less successful when introduced as an aid to organizational efficiency. Doctors have demonstrated an unwillingness to accept such systems into their day to day clinic work. In large part this reluctance relates to a desire to avoid or minimize the standardization of their work and its associated documentation (notably the case notes). Doctors' have the ability to maintain a high degree of indeterminacy in their clinical work (Jamous and Peloille, 1970) and this has direct relevance to the issue of computer-based medical records as has been shown in this chapter. Junior medical staff looked for a degree of standardization in case note structure (of a narrative kind) hospital consultants much prefer the freedom to adopt their own idiosyncratic and particular approaches to case notes. Nonetheless, this particularity of approach does have its own coherent rationale which designers and implementors of computer-based medical records need to take account if they wish to gain routine acceptance. Similarly, such considerations present a challenge to the establishment of medical audit within the new quasi-marketed NHS hospital service. Indeed, the early evidence indicates that medical audit has been embraced by the profession as a system of education and socialization into the profession but little progress has been made in terms of its role as arbiter of medical performance and effectiveness. As for the IT support, this too appears to be under-developed and limited. The conclusion should not be, however, that more computer support will necessarily encourage more medical involvement. The indications are that hospital doctors are concerned to keep medical audit separate from wider hospital systems and would resist or demonstrate extreme apathy towards any such developments.

6 Nurses and computers: technical rationality and emotional labour

Introduction

In this chapter the focus will be on hospital-based nursing computer systems and information technology. Nurses have demonstrated some reticence towards the use of information technology in their work yet they are no 'techno-phobes'. There have always been individuals and groups within the profession more than willing to be actively involved in developing IT systems (e.g. Saba and McCormick, 1996, pp.4-51; Dent et al., 1992, pp.133-4) and who have their own nursing specialist group within the British Computer Society and MEDINFO (e.g. Willis, 1994, p.13; Saba and McCormick, 1996, p.33). Moreover, any reserve of nursing towards IT does not extend to the equipment-embedded technologies used within intensive care and the like (Saba and McCormick, 1986). Why then have nurses demonstrated a degree of resistance to the routine use of computer-based information systems? This is a key question given the current wide-spread introduction of computer-based nurse management information systems as part of the general resource management (RM)policy (Keen and Malby, 1992, pp.867-9; Malby and Clayton, 1994, p.74). This means the nurses will now be expected to use such systems on a daily basis. What will be the implications for nurses and nursing work?

I will argue that the nurses' reservations over information technology relate to three key issues. First, the perceived threat of the new managerialism to the professional status of nursing. Secondly, the continued medical dominance of doctors within the division of labour. Thirdly, the apparent contradiction between the 'emotional labour' (Hochschild, 1983) of bedside care and the technical rationality of computer systems (Strauss, et al., 1983). These issues can also be presented in the form of oppositional binaries as follows:

1. managerialism vs professionalism;
2. medical dominance vs inter-disciplinary teamwork;

3. technological rationality vs emotional labour.

These usefully capture the occupational and organizational tensions within nursing which information technology can exacerbate. All three sets of issues have become particularly apparent with the implementation of resource management (RM) systems but in reality they have a longer history in relation to nurses use of hospital computer systems. Moreover, nurses use a wider range of systems in their work than those that underpin resource management. This chapter explores the range and types of systems used by nurses as well analysing their responses to them.

Structure of the chapter

The chapter starts with an overview of nurses concerns with information technology and distinguishes these as between (a) the main types of nursing systems and (b) systems used by nurses.

Next is a short section that deals with IT for nursing education and research the one area more or less wholly under the control of the profession.

There then follows a treatment of ward-based systems. Here the organizational and occupational dimensions are of particular interest in explaining the nursing responses to their introduction. The section focuses on the Audit Commission's (1992a) report on *Caring Systems*, the influential 'handbook' on ward nursing management and information systems (NMIS) within the National Health Service. Of particular interest is the introduction of care planning systems.

The focus then shifts to those systems that nurses share with other users in the form of multi/inter-disciplinary clinical systems whether as order communications systems (e.g. laboratories and pharmacy), patient administration (PAS) or clinical systems. The main focus here will be on the clinical systems as they are distinct from the ward nursing and management information systems and raise more directly issues of the impact of IT on patient care.

Each section will be concerned with the themes set out in the introduction - i.e. managerialism vs professionalism, medical dominance vs teamwork and technological rationality vs emotional labour - the emphasis, however, will vary from section to section.

Nurses' ambivalence to computer systems

Since the introduction of resource management the official pressure for nurses to adopt computer systems has substantially increased. This encouragement relates primarily to the government's desire for the NHS to control expenditure on nursing and midwifery. This currently stands at just over one third of health authorities' revenue expenditure. It stood at 36 per cent in 1989 of which nearly a half (47 per cent) was for all hospital nursing and midwifery (Audit Commission, 1991, para. 1). The IT strategy for nursing is not simply about reducing the numbers of nurses employed but the centrality of cost reduction within the strategy cannot be underestimated. The drive for cost efficiency, however, is disguised or, more accurately, the organization of nursing has now been changed so that nursing services can be delivered less expensively but, apparently, of better quality. Here the role of the 'named nurse' (Audit Commission, 1991, para. 12), nursing standards and 'skill mix' all play an important part and assumed to require some degree of IT systems support (e.g. Malby and Clayton, 1994, pp.74-5). It is not the intent here to argue that any simplistic de-skilling process is taking place (Braverman, 1974) for the process is far from simple. Nevertheless, the role IT is playing in the re-organization of nursing on acute wards is being perceived by many nurses as a threat to their professionalism.

A North American study recently reported that nurses using computers in their work were 'less negative about their work' (Ngin, Simms and Erbin-Roesemann, 1993, p.127) and that they have a 'positive orientation toward use of computers' (ibid.). The study used a bizarre variant of a job satisfaction measure known as the work excitement tool' (ibid.). In line with the extravagance of the concept 'work excitement' the study also tends to over-emphasize the positive perceptions of nurses in arguing that 'the introductions of computers could ... improve unit morale' (ibid.). The authors acknowledge that there is much evidence to suggest that there are disadvantages as well as advantages to adopting new computer systems (e.g. Hodson and Parker, 1988; Sorenson, 1991). Moreover, they identify and list serious concerns of the North American nurses relating to the new technology:

1. de-skilling
2. undermines the holistic nursing role
3. stress ('burnout').

These are also issues that impinge directly on the hospital nurses expectations and experience of the technology within the NHS more so than the notion of 'excitement' (Rundell, 1991; Keen and Malby, 1992, pp.867-88). At the same time there is also evidence that nursing systems are experienced positively by nurses within UK hospitals (Buchanan, 1993; Kearsley, Little and Wiseman, 1994). Nevertheless, the general position of nurses towards IT and computing can only be described as one of ambivalence. Salvage (1988), in an article appropriately entitled 'The double-edged sword', clearly identified the focus of the concerns when she wrote:

> When health service managers talk about quality and effectiveness, they are often using them as smoke screens for tighter financial control. New nursing management systems built around information technology may be a means of implementing central policy, especially

> fiscal, rather than policy that nurses themselves have developed. (1988, p.65)

Whilst the introduction of resource management is not mentioned directly within the article it is clearly implicit to the argument. More recently Keen and Malby (1992) have also addressed the issue of nursing and IT explicitly in connection with resource management. Their conclusion that the implementation of resource management 'has been a mixed blessing for nurses' (p.869) equally applies to the IT too. The IT corollary of resource management is the computer-based ward nurse management and information system (NMIS) this is not, however, the only variety of nursing information technology available or in use. Computer systems are also being used by nurses for other purposes too. It will be useful to clarify what is meant by nursing systems for it will help us to differentiate between them in terms of the nurses' responses to their introduction and use.

Types of nursing systems

Information technology within nursing can be divided into four main areas of activity:

1. nursing management
2. nursing practice
3. nursing research
4. nursing education.

While nurses commonly express reservations over the introduction of nursing management and nursing practice systems this is not the case with the use of computers for research and education. The uses of computers in these latter areas lie largely (but not entirely) outside the ward. They are neither central to the nursing labour process nor the politics underpinning the social construction of nursing systems generally. Moreover, both research and education are under the control of the profession and not shared with management. I shall start with a brief account of these types of systems.

Computer systems in nursing research and education

Unlike medicine computer applications for nursing education and research have been kept largely separate from the day-to-day work of the wards. Nurses actively involved in education and research have had access to the range of computer applications open to any other academic or clinical researcher. Nursing education within the NHS generally has not played a significant role in increasing general awareness and understanding of IT although this may now be changing. An Institute of Health Services Management survey reported 'a burning need for information-management education' (Willis, 1994, p.14) despite a widespread recognition of its importance within the nurse education establishment. The situation would seem to reflect that which has existed in the US for some time. A national survey carried out there in 1984 revealed a general lack of courses on computer use for nursing. The main emphasis was on word processing and administrative functions with only limited research and computer-aided learning applications being used (Walker, 1986, p.166). Riley (1996, pp.527-73), presents an overview of recent educational applications which indicates that computer developments have predominantly been in the areas of computer-aided learning in the form of Computer Aided Instruction and Interactive Video Instruction (IAV).

McCormick (1986, p.330) listed six major uses of computers as follows:

1. Information retrieval (e.g. CINAHL, MEDLINE)
2. Data processing (e.g. SPSS-X)
3. Graphic displays
4. Database management systems
5. Text editing (i.e. word processing).

In the updated version of the chapter (Saba and McCormick, 1996, pp. 575-616) reference is made to the Internet for on-line communications between researchers. Whilst, spreadsheets and desktop publishing have been added to the researchers armoury to ease problems of analysis and improve the presentation of research findings.

What is not discussed in that chapter but which has emerged as an important focus for nursing research is artificial intelligence (AI) or expert systems. The North American nursing literature has begun to concentrate more than before on IT as a priority for nursing research (Moritz, 1990, pp.111-15) in particular expert systems. Moreover, there has been some interest in marrying nursing theory with information technology to create nursing expert systems (McLaughlin, et al., 1990). However, there does appears to be a major difficulty in adapting 'rule-based' models to nurses' decision-making processes not shared by their medical colleagues (see Chapter 5). There are major difficulties in designing such a system that is capable of providing reasons for its nursing 'advice' (as with any expert system) not least because it is necessary for such systems to include the 'experiential' as well as 'scientific' knowledge which in practice is very difficult to do adequately.

At least three strategies for designing a nursing expert system have been tried. First possibility is to use expert system shells (Jones, 1991). This is the strategy of using a successful medical expert system (e.g. MYCIN) that has been emptied of its previous knowledge content leaving only its basic structure (or shell). Into this shell nursing knowledge can be placed This system is an example of a 'rule-based' approach with the limitations that brings for practical nursing. Nevertheless, by providing an a priori template does reduce the problems associated with capturing the knowledge of the 'experts'. The second strategy has been the adoption of a case-based reasoning approach (Riesbeck and Schank, 1989; Bradburn et al., 1993). This approach is based on standardized care plans. In the example of FLORENCE, a well-advanced prototype being developed in Australia (Bradburn et al., 1993), a new case/patient is first allocated to a standard case as determined by the medical diagnosis (as would be normal practice with care plans) which would be retrieved from the case files (again as with care plans). Only unexplained features of the case will be reviewed by the system in consultation with the user (Bradburn et al., 1993, p.22). Its case-based orientation reflects nursing practice and in computer terms is a hybrid of expert and data-base system. The nursing diagnostic level provides the expert component elicited by inputting the 'major defining characteristics' (p.23) of the patients' cases which can be weighted on a scale of 1 to 5.

The data-base level provides the third strategy for overcoming the limitations of 'rule based' expert systems methodology. Here it is the case library that provides the data-base (of cases). It is from this that any variations from standard cases can identified and included in the drawing up fully customized care plans. This type of system has the advantage of paralleling a decision process with which nurses are familiar (i.e. care planning).

Expert systems have the advantage of providing a particular focus for research and development that attempts to link the experiential and scientific knowledge bases of nursing as a contribution to nursing theory. Moreover, it offers an opportunity for more nurse researchers to specialize in information systems and computing work entirely independent of medical dominance or managerial interests. Expert systems, however, are unlikely to become a standard application on the wards for the foreseeable future. Its main role is likely remain in the area of nursing research although the relation between specialist care and diagnoses and research may well prove to be a two way process. Part of the reason for this continued research focus relates to current interest in the use of computers to aid the understanding of nursing theory, reasoning and diagnosis (McLaughlin et al., 1990; Moritz, 1990; Jones, 1991; Rios et al., 1991). Another reason, however, is that nursing practice on the ward has proven resistant to computerization. It is to this topic I now turn although this time the theme is the relation between nursing practice and ward management and the implications this may or may not have for nurses' professional status and the nature of their work.

Ward management and practice

Since the introduction of resource management the pressure for nurses to adopt computer systems has substantially increased. This encouragement relates primarily to the government's desire for the NHS to control pay expenditure on nursing and midwifery. In 1988-89 the cost was almost £5 billion or 36 per cent of health authorities' revenue expenditure. The figure represents nearly a half (47 per cent) of all NHS salary costs (Audit Commission, 1991, para. 1). This covers all nursing areas including Community and Mental Illness and Handicap. 'Adult Acute Wards', however, is the single most expensive category accounting for 26 per cent of the nursing and midwifery salaries (ibid.). While it is the case that doctors earn substantially more than nurses the overall pay costs for the latter are more than three times as much. Hence the policy concern to control nursing costs has led to a rise in managerialism within nursing. This in turn has raised worries within the profession that the recent organizational reforms may threaten a degree of de-professionalization. The actual policies pursued by government and the nursing profession, however, are more complex than that. The combination of skill mix on the wards and restructuring of nursing has given rise to a clear distinction between professional 'core' and an army of nursing health care auxiliaries. Computer-based nursing systems have been seen to have an important part to play in managing the new staffing arrangements.

In 1992 the Audit Commission published its report entitled *Caring Systems* (1992a) on IT for nurses. Unlike many other Audit reports it was not intended to be a critical scrutiny of current shortcomings as, for instance, was the case with the HISS programme (1990b, reported in Computer Weekly, 1990b). Instead the *Caring Systems* report was designed as a 'handbook ... to help project nurses and others choose and implement a ward nursing management and information system' (p.1). It was the second such handbook published by the Audit Commission. The first being *Making Time for Patients* (Audit Commission, 1992b) which was concerned with identifying ways of disseminating good nursing practice and improving the quality of patient care (1992a, para 1). Both were the consequence of the earlier report *The Virtue of Patients* (1991) which recommended an agenda of action of senior hospital managers to improve nursing services within the new organizational arrangements and resource management (1992a, para 11). The *Caring Systems* handbook was confined to dealing with ward-based nursing systems but included consideration of their potential role for quality assurance, audit and research (e.g. para 40).

The authors recognised that nurses would often be using systems other than specifically nursing ones including, clinical information systems and ward ordering & communications systems. The report subscribed to the ideal that 'information systems should be based on the individual patient and be used by all health care staff, irrespective of profession, in order to support the provision of high quality, collaborative, seamless care.' (ibid., para 2; see Fig. 6.1). In many ways the separation of 'nursing' from other hospital systems is an artificial distinction. Computerized nursing management systems may be included within a wider networked hospital system (e.g. HISS) and may well include (or interface with) a ward ordering and communication component (module), certain patient administration (PAS) functions and/or be linked to payroll or a case-mix management system

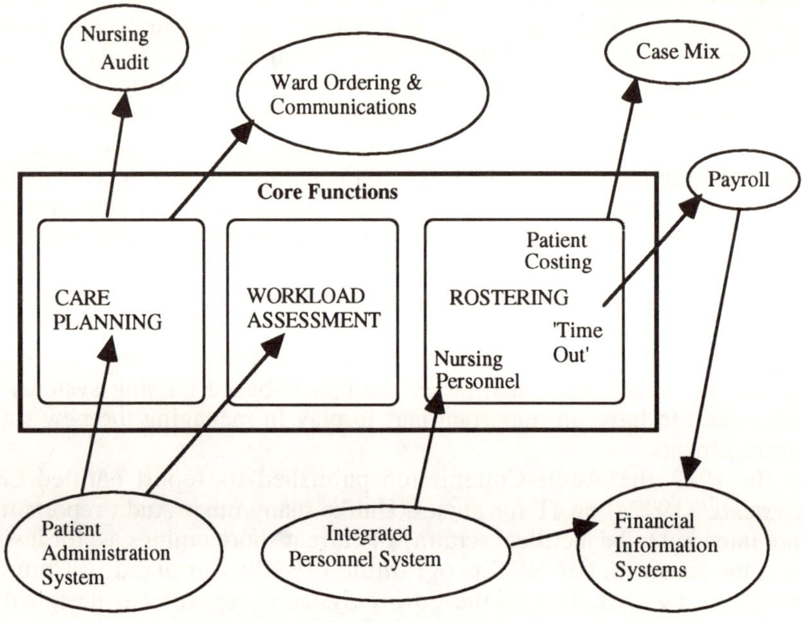

Figure 6.1 Ward nursing management and information systems

(Source: Audit Commission: 1992a, p. 5)

(CMMS) (Paras. 9 -10). Instead, as the 'handbook' notes, '[g]reat impetus was given to ... nursing by the Department of Health's timetable for ... Resource Management.' (para. 11) and hospitals were pressurized to order nursing systems by the second year of resource management funding and implement them by the end of the third year (ibid.). This time scale limits the degree of integration initially possible between nursing and other systems as well as pressurizing nurses to adopt a technology many find threatening to their central rationale; patient care. The handbook attempts to negotiate a path between these constraints and offer advice on how to achieve working nursing systems without compromising nursing care and which can be integrated into broader based hospital systems.

The handbook identifies three core functions for computer-based nursing systems (Fig. 6.1):

1. Care planning
2. Workload assessment

Table 6.1 Use of nurse management systems in major acute general hospitals

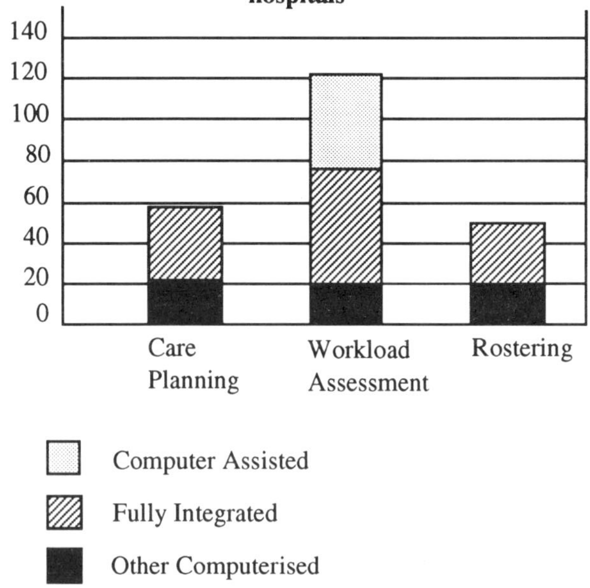

(Source: Audit Commission (1992a) p. 5)

3. Rostering.

These may be integrated although this does not appear to be a common practice. According to the Audit Commission's own estimates workload assessment is the most commonly computer-based or assisted activity and care planning the least (see Table 6.1). The only generalization that can be made is that the distribution and usage of these systems is very variable. For instance, in the ten hospitals studied in detail by the handbook's authors four had introduced computer-assisted care planning on some wards, four had introduced workload assessment systems and three computerized rostering. Only one hospital was making full use of an integrated hospital system (para 10). Two recent articles on nursing systems (Buchanan, 1993; Thompson and Marshall, 1993) suggest that they are capable of being introduced and used to improve quality of care and reduce costs as well as being positively accepted by the users. The first to be considered is Thompson and Marshall's report on the introduction of the Crescendo ward management system at the Royal Hallamshire Hospital. The strategy adopted was one using the system to reduce the administrative and managerial component of the nursing work. In care planning the aim was to reduce the time spent on drawing up care plans per patient. The manual method was calculated to take 18 minutes to create and 6 minutes to update. This compared with the automated system which reduced the average time to 3.9 minutes to create and between 1.7-2.6 minutes to update. The care plans component of the system produces the workload figures automatically and translates these into the required skill mix for each ward. Preparation of rosters can, additionally, take into account sickness, annual leave, transfers (etc.) to produce a better match between staff and workload. This in turn is seen to contribute to a general improvement of quality. The technicist optimism of the Thompson and Marshall report (1993) is not shared by Buchanan (1993) who points to the problems of project management in the implementation of computerized care planning. In this report there is much more emphasis on the computer system (GALAXY) supporting the 'chosen model of nursing' (p.38).

The contrast between the two approaches is less about the systems than about the organization and control of nursing work. The concern to drive down the time involved in care planning and to use of this data more for nursing management purposes could lead to the situation as described by a sister elsewhere (Keen and Malby, 1992, p.868) where 'the ward staff have [gone] from working hard to produce excellent care plans hand-written, to printing trash'. It is the care of the patient that is the primary rationale of care plans not rostering and workload assessments.

Depending on the type of ward pre-printed or word processed templates may be more appropriate and less expensive method (Audit Commission, 1992, para. 51). The current strategy of automating care plans is an equivocal one in terms of whether the emphasis is on providing information to improve nursing practice or gathering information for more effective management control. The two are not necessarily incompatible or even undesirable but only when the distinctions are clear and well understood. This does not appear to be the case of care planning systems and nurse management systems. Keen and Malby (1992), in their discussion of IT (in the context of resource management), conclude that nurses' experiences of ward based IT has been highly equivocal. These authors relate this ambivalent situation to the fact that while resource management seemed to offer the opportunity for nurses to play a more central role in the management process. In the event, nursing power was not strengthened and there was concern that nursing practice was adversely affected (ibid., p.869). In part this was seen as a consequence of '[s]enior nurses ... often impos[ing] computer systems on ward staff' (ibid., p.869). This whole set of inter-related issues of IT and nursing power and practice also has an important gender dimension. The profession is predominantly female and historically was located in a 'handmaiden' relation to the dominant medical profession (e.g. Davies, 1992, pp.234-5). The gendered subordination for nurses is of a different order, however, to that of the female health service manager or clerk (Davies and Rosser, 1986) for unlike them the profession as a whole is gendered female. The senior grades of nursing are 70 per cent female. This means, of course, that 30 per cent of them are male which is an over-representation of the species for they only constitute 10 per cent of the profession as a whole (Davies, 1992, p.229). Nevertheless, it is still a much higher number than in medicine or management. The problem for nurses is that the historically gendered nature of their profession not only has weakened their power position within the health service but also their organizational ability to counter this (Davies, 1992). This relates directly to the contention of Keen and Malby (1992) that resource management and the associated IT systems had initially appeared to offer an opportunity for nurse empowerment but had failed to deliver. Their conclusion is that this relates to nurses being poor at 'play[in] the management game for which [they found] them ill prepared.'(p.864).

It would appear that nursing is subject to the full range of labour process strategies identified by Child (1985):

1. elimination of direct labour
2. contracting (bank nurses)
3. polyvalence
4. degradation of jobs.

Ward nurse management information systems may not be the direct cause of all of these but these systems do have a role of closely monitoring the impact of the strategies. Thus, the more tightly scheduled work rosters and skill mix the smaller the numbers of qualified nurses required on the wards which adds up to (1) elimination of direct labour. This is so even if the actual numbers of qualified staff does not decline so long as more patients are being treated more quickly. This may lead to more reliance on (2) contracting of agency nurses to deal with temporary or new increases in demand or simply to cover for annual and study leave. In addition, there is a clearly identifiable trend towards extending the hospital nursing role in order to cover tasks and responsibilities previously carried out by doctors. The introduction of triage nurses in accident and emergency units (Read and George, 1994) is an example of this type of (3) polyvalence strategy. This 'in the French sense of the term, denot[es] a situation in which workers perform, or at least are available to perform, a range of tasks which cut across or extend traditional skill and job boundaries' (Child, 1985, p.125). Whether this will mean the development will lead on to the development of a genuine nurse practitioner role within the hospital sector (e.g. Fagin, 1992) is far from certain but it will mean that for qualified nurses there is the real opportunity to avoid the worst aspects of (4) degradation of jobs. This, however, is largely because the new nursing structures have brought about a more stratified occupation with only the upper echelons avoiding the routinization of their work (e.g. via standardized care plans) and maintaining an outer bastion against a general de-professionalization. Nursing professionals are increasingly being involved in the management and organization of patient care as distinct from its delivery. This raises a basic ontological question as to the nature of nursing; is it the management and care of patients or the management of the management and care of patients? Certainly current trends point to the latter. In which case the caring role of nursing would appear to be increasingly peripheralized. This aspect is best examined here through a discussion of clinical computer systems which are directly concerned with the delivery of patient and medical care.

Clinical computing systems

In broad terms, nursing is differentiated from medicine in terms of its focus on patient care (rather than 'cure'). This in large part reflects an ambivalence in the nurses' occupational status as between professional autonomy and doctors 'handmaiden' (Davies, 1992, pp.234-5). One important aspect of this ambivalence concerns the relative autonomy of the core activities of nursing relating to patient care. These activities include components which Hochschild defined as 'emotional labour' (1983) and Strauss et al. (1982, 1985) as 'sentimental work'. This aspect of nursing care is particularly relevant to our understanding of clinical computer systems. In this section the focus is on the introduction of one such system within two hospitals renal units. The study will provide a more detailed analysis of nursing work, variations in nursing/medical division of labour and the importance of the caring/emotional aspects of patient care.

Clinical computing: The renal case study

Renal units exist primarily to dialyse patients with end stage renal failure (ESRF) and to train them to dialyse themselves. An important aspect of the care of renal patients is the regularly monitoring and recording of their condition by the nurses and doctors. In consequence, the renal units possess an extensive set of records on each of their dialysis patients. This section reports on a study of two renal units and the consequences of the introduction of a computerized patient data system. This system was designed to ease the burden on the nurses of manually maintaining the patient records as well as improve the access and analysis of the clinical data for the doctors. The concern here is not whether the system was accepted or rejected but how it came to be used and why. Using an approach informed by labour process analysis, this study demonstrates the ways in which the clinical division of labour 'shaped' the ways in which the computer system was used and not the other way around.

The clinical computing system was designed to automate the collation and presentation of clinical data in a manner that emulated the clinic record. This document has been the subject of some sociological interest. The concern, however, has related primarily to the doctor-patient relations (see Chapter 5) whereas the particular concern here is the organization of the inter/multi-disciplinary clinic work. It will be argued that variations in the acceptability and usage of the computer system are to be understood in terms of different medical rationales of the consultants which are consequent, in large part, on the different histories of the units. Moreover, these rationales have consequences for the organization and control of nursing.

The field work was carried out over a three year period (1983-86) in two hospitals in the English midlands. The first renal unit had facilities only for haemo-dialysis while the second provided more than one form of dialysis therapy and had facilities for carrying out kidney transplants as well. Hence the first unit will be referred to as the Haemo Unit and the second, the Dialysis Unit.

The Renal Computer System and its consequences

The Renal Computer System (a fictitious name) was a renal patient database system designed to aid the accurate and timely collection, collation and presentation of clinical and related data (concerning administrative, dietetics and social work records). The general objective of the system was to enable the doctors and nurses to better monitor the well-being of renal patients than possible was the case with the traditional hand-written clinic records. It was also the case that the consultants intended the system to provide them with facilities to support medical audit and research activities.

The System was bought as a 'package' at the behest of the renal consultants and with the intention of the Regional Health Authority that it would be installed and made operational with the minimum of technical support. It was implemented at the 5 renal units within the region with the support of a single computer specialist. A level of technical support that was inadequate and led to delays and frustrations in the implementation and development of the system.

What is particularly interesting is that the introduction of a standard computer 'package' into the two units reported on here led to a marked variation in its utilization and the responses of the nurses (and doctors). This illuminated (i.e. made explicit) the character of the organizational and social relations between nurses, doctors and dialysis patients. At the first unit it was the medical staff and senior nurses who liked the system and directly used it in their day-to-day work. The nurses directly involved in dialysing and training patients, however, found the system burdensome. In marked contrast, at the second renal unit the nurses found the system a direct aid to their work and it was the consultants who did not like it. In order to explain the reasons for these differences the nature of renal work and its organization will be elaborated in order to demonstrate that it is the social and organizational processes that principally determine the consequences of technological innovation and not the other way around.

End stage renal failure and dialysis treatment

Before progressing further with details of the introduction of the computer system some explanation as to the nature of renal dialysis is necessary as this constitutes the basic work activity of the renal units. Dialysis patients suffer from end stage renal failure (ESRF). They are kept alive, and reasonably healthy, through the regular dialysis of their blood. Without dialysis, or a kidney transplant a patient would die within one or two weeks (Gallagher, 1976, p.64). Many patients are trained by the nurses to dialyse themselves at home, this not only gives the patients a degree of autonomy it also relieves the pressure on the units and permits them to take on new patients. Not all patients, however, are able to dialyse at home both for social and medical reasons. These travel to hospital for regular haemo-dialysis on a renal unit.

Renal dialysis essentially takes one of two forms, haemo-dialysis or peritoneal dialysis. Haemo-dialysis involves the patient's blood being pumped through an artificial kidney whereby, through a process of osmosis and filtration, the patient's blood is cleansed of urea and its electrolyte balance is maintained in an approximation of natural kidney function (ibid.). This procedure is normally carried out twice or three times a week for 3-6 hours. New patients, normally, have first to undergo minor surgery so an artery and a vein in the fore-arm can be conjoined to form a fistula large enough to provide access for connecting (via needles and tubing) to the artificial kidney within the haemo dialysis machine.

Peritoneal dialysis systems, on the other hand, exploit the naturally occurring osmotic quality of the peritoneum to cleanse the patient's blood of toxic material. The most common peritoneal technique is that known as Continuous Ambulatory Peritoneal Dialysis (CAPD). With this method the patient's abdominal cavity is loaded with an appropriate quantity of dialysate which is changed about every four hours during the patient's waking life via a plastic (Tenchoff) tube which passes through the abdominal wall.

At the time of the research the senior consultant at the Haemo Unit was committed to haemo-dialysis on the grounds that it was a tried and tested technique whereas CAPD was a relatively new system that had been dogged by problems of peritoneal infections. By contrast, the consultants at the Dialysis Unit favoured the newer method of CAPD as their 'treatment of choice' on the grounds that it (a) was a more 'natural' and 'gentle' process than haemo-dialysis, (b) the dietary restrictions were less onerous for the patient and, importantly, (c) it took less time to teach the patients the procedure (usually no more than two weeks compared to a minimum of six weeks for haemo-dialysis). This meant that more patients could be trained within the same period of time compared with haemo-dialysis. The preferences of the consultants at the two hospitals to the two types of dialysis reflected underlying difference in their general approach to the

Table 6.2 Dialysis patient numbers (Haemo Unit)

Type of patient		No.
Under training		10
Home dialysis		31
*Unit patients**		23
	Total	64

* Unit patients were those patients who were unable to haemo-dialyse at home for various reasons.

management of chronic renal failure and had implications for the division of labour within the two renal units. This in turn had important implications for the ways in which the nursing staff on the two units adapted to the Renal Computer System.

A central activity of all renal units is the regular monitoring of patients' haematological, biochemical and clinical profiles for this data forms a central plank of the doctors' clinical management. This means there is a data-base of considerable size held on each patient which, in turn, presents practical problems of storage, access and analysis. It was these problems that led the renal consultants search for a computer-based solution. Before discussing the system, however, it will be useful to describe the way the two units were organized.

The Renal Units: Haemo Unit

The Haemo unit was established in 1970, initially as a satellite of another renal unit. At the time of the research there were two consultant physicians (with a special interest in renal medicine) and one registrar routinely involved with the care of the dialysis patients. The renal unit had two small wards (containing reclining armchairs) for dialysis and training sufficient for 8 patients at any one time. The unit staff were responsible for 64 dialysis patients (see Table 6.2). The total number of dialysis patients was not far short of half the number (119 patients) at other unit (see Table 6.4). Most patients were expected to become sufficiently well trained in haemo-dialysis that they could routinely dialyse at home. This was the responsibility of the

Table 6.3 Nursing staff (Haemo Unit)

Grade	No.
Nursing Officer	1
Sisters	2
Enrolled and Registered Nurses	9
Auxiliaries	2
Total	14

nurses of which there were fourteen, exactly half the number at the second unit (see Table 6.3 and 6.5). The nurses at this unit were rostered to cover two shifts, early and late. The nursing officer had organized the work of the nurses broadly in line with the criteria of the nursing process (Walton, 1987). In principle, this meant that each nurse was individually responsible for the dialysis and training of specific patients on her shift. Dialysis training at this unit was judged by the staff (both nursing and medical) to involve more than patients learning to carry out the dialysis procedures. They had also to become accustomed to the necessity of living with the discipline of haemodialysis. For the nurses this involved a mix of emotional labour and sentimental work (Hochschild, 1983; Strauss et al., 1982, 1985).

The training period, invariably in excess of the minimum six weeks, gave time for the patient, and the patient's family, to adapt to the regime. This aspect of the nursing work is classifiable as sentimental work (Strauss et al., 1982; 1985) and more particular the sub-types, composure and identity work. Composure work, involved 'helping, or enjoining patients to keep their composure' (1985, p.136) whilst undergoing dialysis and identity work is a matter 'of getting ... persons to face the realities of their physical conditions and prepare them for their post-hospital lives' (1985, p.138). This particular inter-weaving of technical training and emotional adaptation to the haemodialysis regime can also be analyzed in terms of emotional labour (Hochschild, 1983). That is to say, nurses were expected to respond to the patient in a way which is personal to both of them even though it develops and is shaped by the clinical labour process (James, 1988, pp.16-17). This is an example of the social construction of emotions (Fineman, 1994, pp.80-3). There are clear parallels between the two concepts of sentimental work and emotional labour. They both relate to the role the nurse play in befriending a patient so s/he may be trained up that much quicker than would otherwise be the case. There is a difference, however, and it is of some significance.

Sentimental work is a set of techniques available to the nurses and subject to their control. They decide which technique to use and when to apply it. The concept stems from the social interactionist perspective which concentrates on the inter-personal and inter-group relations rather than the structured relations within the division of labour (or the organization and control of the nurses). Emotional labour, on the other hand, focuses more on the asymmetrically structured power relations within the hospital. Staff are expected to display particular emotions so the work can be done more efficiently. Fineman's (1994) example of McDonald's fast food restaurants could be said also to apply to renal dialysis nursing for just as the counter staff at McDonald's are expected to display 'sincerity, enthusiasm, confidence and a sense of humour' (Boas and Chain, 1976) so to do nurses no matter what they really feel like.

Within the Haemo unit there was a considerable emphasis put on the emotional labour aspect of the nursing work. The senior medical and nursing staff would decide the strategy (an example of 'sentimental work') while the nurses would have to carry out the work (i.e. emotional labour). If a patient did not respond to the 'befriending' approach, however, then they might undergo other emotional processes associated with identity work such as ostracism (see 'The case of the oven cooked chips', see Box 6.1). It was this application of emotional labour that helped ensure that the maximum numbers of patients were trained in home haemo-dialysis. In contrast, the emotional content of nursing work was not nearly so strongly emphasized at the other unit and this difference contributed significantly to the different responses of the nurses at the two units.

Alongside the emotional labour and sentimental work the nurses had the technical task of recording patient data. Blood pressure, temperatures and weights were recorded at the time of dialysis, while biochemical and haematological data was collected monthly. At the Haemo Unit the collation of this data was carried out by the senior nurses only (i.e. nursing officer and sisters) to leave the nursing staff free to develop their emotional skills and concentrate on the dialysis and training of patients. This was not the case at the second unit.

The organization of the sentimental work was further reinforced through the weekly case conferences which involved senior nursing staff, doctors and others. The subjects covered at these meetings were as follows:

1. Any problems (medical, social or psychological) relating to the patients' chronic ESRF status.

2. patient training.

3. matters relating to the installation of a haemo-dialysis machine in the patient's home.

Box 6.1 The case of the oven cooked chips

A patient in his twenties had not been adhering to his diet. This was evident from the results of his monthly blood tests. This lack of dietary discipline was seen as a sign of his immaturity, 'He will have to toe the line and grow up' (Registrar). The nursing sister reported that the patient saw the unit's rules relating to dialysis and the dietary restrictions as arbitrary and had failed to become sufficiently proficient to carry out haemo-dialysis at home. The healthcare team decided to adopt a two pronged strategy of reward and social isolation, if the patient could get his potassium level down to a medically tolerable level he would be rewarded with oven cooked chips being included in his diet. But to accompany the 'carrot' there was to be a 'stick' and the other part of the strategy was that this patient would be socially isolated when he was dialysing on the unit. This ostracism was to continue until his dietary discipline had improved and he had consciously set about learning to dialyse effectively on his own. This decision was taken during the August and in following December at one of the 'Monday Morning Meetings' one of the sisters was able to report that he was now 'very co-operative'.

Virtually all discussions of the dialysis patients started with an examination of the clinical and laboratory data initially via the patients' clinic records. Only when these had been found to be inconclusive would non-medical factors be considered. Nevertheless, many of the discussions at these meetings related to matters not strictly medical. One case which illustrates well the way the meetings worked and co-ordinated the orchestration of emotional labour was the 'case of the oven cooked chips' (see Box 6.1). Clearly at this renal unit there was considerable emphasis sentimental work in order to gain and maintain patient discipline as the means of delivering good patient care. The medical and nursing staff, with the support of the dietician and other occupations, would attempt with some success to bring about behavioural changes through surveillance and the application of sentimental work. This orientation of the unit had strong resonance of Foucault's (1977) analysis of the panopticon a point that will be developed later. This orientation was not shared by the second unit.

Renal Units: Dialysis and transplant

The Dialysis Unit had been established in the late sixties, a little before the Haemo Unit, by the professor of nephrology. The unit was designed to

Table 6. 4 Dialysis patients numbers (Dialysis Unit)

Type of patient		No.
Haemo-dialysed at home		60
Haemo-dialysed on the unit		12
Patients on CAPD at home		40
Patients on training (CAPD)		6
Patients on CCPD at home		1
	Total	119

incorporate all aspects of end stage renal failure nursing and most of their medical care. It was an altogether larger unit than the Haemo Unit both in terms of staff employed and patients treated. The unit contained a number of individual rooms and small wards (3-4 beds), plus one larger ward (8 beds). In total the unit had 18 beds available for inpatients. Patients undergoing transplantation were cared for on the unit as were chronic renal patients under-going investigations or treatment requiring an inpatient stay. At the time of the research there were a total of 119 patients (Table 6.4). This unit offered three types of dialysis therapy:

1. haemo-dialysis
2. continuous ambulatory peritoneal dialysis (CAPD)
3. continuous cyclic peritoneal dialysis (CCPD).

The last variety is a variation on CAPD but the changes of dialysate take place at night while the patient is at rest. It is useful for people who cannot have access to a clean area where they can change their dialysate under sterile conditions during the day.

There were two consultant nephrologists and one transplant surgeon. In addition, there was one senior registrar, one registrar and two senior house officers (SHOs). As with the Haemo Unit the consultants also held general medical clinics where the junior medical staff also assisted. The majority of the doctors' work was directly related to renal medicine (excepting the transplant surgeon who was principally employed as a urologist). In contrast to the practice at the Haemo Unit, the day to day medical work associated with this unit was wholly delegated to the senior registrar which was to prove to be a factor of some significance when considering the consultants ultimate antipathy towards the Renal Computer System.

Table 6.5 Nursing staff (Dialysis Unit)

Grade	No.
Associate Director of Nursing Services (ADNS)	1
Ward Sisters	2
Enrolled and Registered Nurses	24
Auxiliary	1
Total	28

Nursing on the unit was headed by an Assistant Director of Nursing Services (ADNS) this was an administrative post which carried responsibilities for the organization of nursing work throughout the hospital. The day to day management of nursing work was the responsibility of the two nursing sisters. The full complement of nursing staff was twenty-eight (Table 6.5). This was considerably larger than the Haemo Unit which functioned with fourteen nurses (Table 6.2). Yet the difference in numbers of patients between the two units was less than might be anticipated given these staffing levels.

The Haemo Unit had 10 dialysis patients being trained and 23 who dialysed on the unit (Table 6.2). By contrast, the Dialysis Unit had only 6 patients undergoing training and a further 12 patients who dialysed at the unit (Table 6.4). There were, however, 101 patients dialysing at home (haemo-dialysis, CAPD and CCPD) which was a much higher figure than the Haemo Unit's total of 31. All these patients required regular monitoring and investigation. By comparison to the previous unit, there was considerably more data-processing and rather less patient-processing work.

While the nurses considered themselves to be organized according to nursing process principles, dialysis and patient training were not given as central a role as was the case at the other unit and less emphasis was placed on sentimental work than at the Haemo Unit. Instead, all the nurses (excepting the auxiliary) were responsible for maintaining and collating the patient data records and providing assistance at clinics and meetings. These tasks are not central to nursing process which is, in essence, concerned with patient-centred nursing care (Walton, 1986, p.13). The nurse duties (other than the haemo-dialysis of patients) were organized on a group basis either on a 6 month rotation or according to the time of day. The duties on the six month rota were as follows:

1. CAPD patient training;

2. clinic work (nurses acted as receptionists and provided the doctors with the patients' clinic files as required);

3. 'bloods' and tissue typing (the organization of the collection and dispatch of blood - and urine samples - for monthly assessment and checking for transplantation purposes);

4. ward and graph rounds (nurses allocated to these meetings were responsible for supplying the doctors with the medical records or patients charts).

Tasks 2-4 were to be computerized which meant that the routine work of the nurses was more directly affected than was the case at the Haemo Unit. The computerization impact was to prove to be equally great on the 'time of day' organization of work. This referred to the entry and presentation of clinic and laboratory data. Each nurse was individually responsible for the entry of patient's dialysis-related data (e.g. weight, blood pressure). The collation of this data was organized collectively. The sister would allocate the task to a group of nurses on an ad hoc basis every evening. The laboratory results would also be entered into the clinic records at the same time. Then, uniquely, within the health region the nurses would draw up graphs of all this patient data. These graphs were referred to as the 'charts' and were checked each month at the Graph Round by the senior registrar. The Renal Computer System was to computerize this whole process.

The Graph Round constituted the central rationale for the nurses collating and charting the patients' laboratory and clinical data. The monthly meeting was held in the patients' lounge. Here all the hand-drawn graphs completed by the nurses throughout the month were checked by the senior registrar. S/he would always be assisted by one of the junior doctors and three, sometimes, four nurses. The procedure would be as follows. One nurse would hand a 'chart' (i.e. graph) to the registrar for scrutiny, the second, the relevant medical record. The third, the sister on duty, noted down any changes in the patient's dialysis regime or related treatment so far as it affected the nursing staff. If the senior registrar was satisfied with the patient's chart s/he would endorse the case-notes with the acronym 'GROK' (being short for 'Graph OK.'). If that was not the case then s/he would enter details of the investigations or therapies that were to be pursued. The meeting was, in fact, an example of medical audit (i.e. a chart review) (Roemer and Friedman, 1971; Dent, 1995a), although no doctor seemed to be aware of this fact despite being specifically asked about the subject. Following computerization the graph round used visual display terminals (VDUs) instead of the graphs and took two to three times longer to complete with the same number of staff. Unlike the Haemo Unit there was no inter-disciplinary meeting to discuss dialysis patients and their management.

Box 6.2 The case of the miner and his beer

There was a patient, a miner, that earned himself a special respect among the doctors because of his ability to 'work the [dialysis] system'. Unlike many recalcitrant dialysis patients, he did not reject the system but utilized the technology of haemo-dialysis to, 'dialyse right down, then go down the miner's club for [a few] pints' (Senior Registrar). This miner, with hedonistic intent, had developed his own technique of first dialysing himself until he was 'as dry as a bone' (ibid.). He would then go out for his social evening with his mates. On returning he would haemo-dialyse once again this time to remove the excess fluids.

Patient training was wholly the nurses' affair and there was little attempt to adopt any kind of inter-disciplinary approach to these patients this was so even, as in the case of the Haemo Unit, in attempting to discipline the recalcitrant. There was even some evidence, among the doctors at least, of a certain admiration for the independence of these particular patients. It was their view that patients who failed to dialyse regularly, or sufficiently long enough, or were guilty of dietary indiscretions would cause only themselves discomfort. The probability that these patients were increasing the medical risks to themselves was not seen as sufficient reason to be interventionist beyond giving advice. One consultant expressed the view that 'patients rarely kill themselves because of ill-discipline' and this would seem to have justified a generally tolerant attitude to patient management and well illustrated by the case of the 'Miner and his Beer' (Box 6.2). This case illustrates the contrast in styles of medical management between the two renal units. The Haemo Unit team would view this patient as requiring re-education involving extensive sentimental work particularly on the part of the nurses (as in the case of the 'oven cooked chips') whereas the Dialysis Unit medical staff did not. The consultants there interpreted their role in the care of dialysis patients far more narrowly, limited, virtually, to supervising the junior doctors. Unlike their colleagues at the Haemo Unit, these consultants did not recognise an important role for emotional labour and precluded its consideration in the management of patients.

The computer as panopticon

Clearly, from the accounts of the workings of the two renal units, a central activity of both was the surveillance of dialysis patients to ensure, as far as was possible, their continued well-being. To this end the patients' metabolism was made virtually 'transparent' to the view of the doctors, nurses and others through the medium of the clinic records or 'charts'. This meant that any patient who failed to remain faithful to their dialysis and dietary regime would find their transgressions recorded indelibly in their clinical records and pointed out to them when they next attended clinic. In this respect these patients were subject to a discipline paralleling that of the panopticon (Foucault, 1977; see also Lyon, 1988, pp.98-9). The exercise of that discipline, however, differed considerably between the two units. The consultants at the Haemo Unit had as a core rationale for the introduction of the computer system the improved surveillance of dialysis patients in order to exercise more effective control (discipline) over the patients and their condition. This was less the case with the Dialysis Unit. Here the consultants' prime concern was to develop the computer system as an aid medical research and audit.

The Renal Computer System: Outcomes

Having described and compared the two renal units it is now possible to address the question what were the consequences of the introduction of the Renal Computer System?

(i) The Haemo Unit

One of the computer systems main uses was to display patient data at the weekly inter-disciplinary case meetings. Data was principally entered by a newly appointed part-time computer clerk although the nurses were intended to enter data when the clerk was not on the unit. The consultants used the system directly in clinic to review patient data and in the case of the senior consultant the system was also used as an aid for patient education.

> I think (the computer graphs are) especially valuable because you can show the patients (in clinic) their own results on the (VDU) screen ... and they can see immediately ... where alterations in their treatment ... or diet, etc. have produced visible changes in their blood results I think this has an important educational value ...

The registrar also made any regular use of the computer system. He established himself as the 'in-house' computer specialist to whom the nurses, as well as other doctors, turned to for assistance.

The situation with the nurses was far more ambivalent. The senior nurses benefited most directly from the introduction of the system. Their previous chore of collating and recording patient related data was now carried out by the computer clerk. Furthermore, the presentation of this data on the VDU screen was found to be easier to interpret by the senior nursing staff than was previously the case with the manual system. As one of them explained: 'before, each patient, as their results came back, I had to "pick through" [several different slips of paper] I was recording everywhere, four or five times ... Now at the end of each month, I can literally spend half an hour just "flicking" through each patients results ... on the screen ... I just take "notes" on what I have to act on and that's it'. The nursing staff, on the other hand, found the system of little value. They still had to complete the recording of dialysis data and had little need to access data routinely. As one exasperated nurse explained: 'We are still doing ... everything as before. I thought it would stop us having to do the nursing [record]. I hoped it would stop us from having to do all these [dialysis record sheets] every day'. There were, in addition, facilities for presenting summarised textual information on patients in chronological order. It was the nursing officer and sisters who were responsible for designing these 'events screens' as they are known and teaching the nursing staff how to enter the data themselves. The 'screens' were thought, by all the nurses, to be of no benefit to them given the extra time and effort involved given that the information was already written up in the nursing record (a document the nurses believed they were legally required to maintain). This situation contrasted markedly with the situation at the Dialysis Unit.

(ii) The Dialysis Unit

The computer system was introduced at the Dialysis Unit a few months later than at the Haemo Unit. The responses of the nurses and doctors were markedly different to that found at the Haemo Unit reflecting the contrasting medical rationales of the two units. The entry of dialysis patient data was carried out by the nurses who found the system a general improvement on the previous manual system for it saved them the work of drawing up the charts for each patient. In the words of one of the unit sisters 'its easier, a tremendous improvement on the (hand-written) graphs'.

The junior doctors also found the computer system of benefit and in a way that contrasted markedly with the arrangements at the Haemo Unit. Here 'events screens' were maintained on all patients by the nurses. On these 'screens' were recorded all the medically significant events in a patient's medical career. The junior doctors found this facility a very useful source of patient information, equating to a medical record summary. These events screens were much more readily accessible than the medical records, being literally available at the 'touch of a button'.

> [The events screen] speeded things up, especially in terms of extracting someone's 'previous renal history' from the computer rather than the 'notes' ... If people were coming in ... that I didn't know I would .. go through the events records [screens] to see what was going on with them (Junior Doctor)

The availability of this facility was pointed out to each successive generation of junior doctors by the nursing staff, who were in practice responsible for showing these doctors how to use the system.

The consultants were, by contrast, very critical of the system. They would have liked a system which was better able to analyze aggregate (rather than individual) patient data for medical audit and research purposes. The system as it was implemented was unable to do this and the regional computer staff failed to develop these facilities.

Turning now to the use made of the computer system at meetings and clinics. The raison d'être of the Renal Computer System at this unit was the monthly Graph Round. Here the nursing staff operated two VDUs terminals to access the graphs. There had to be two VDUs as the computer's response time was very slow (especially when compared to the manual method of unrolling large 'charts'); one VDU for patients' weights and blood pressures the other for their biochemistry and haematological results. By alternating between the two VDUs the procedure was speeded up, but the round still took approximately twice as long as had been the case with the hand-drawn 'charts'. Whereas previously the Graph Round had only occupied one morning a month immediately following computerization the meeting had to be extended over two half days. Nevertheless, this extra cost in time, according to the senior registrar, was more than compensated by the system's benefits described in the following terms.

> [Firstly] the computer enables me to look at the patients in more detail (than previously) because of the way the data is presented by the computer, particularly the graphics ... [Secondly], any 'results' that are put down wrongly are more obvious on the computer system than they were on the (manual) chart system and easier to spot. [Thirdly] ... it is less time-consuming for the nurses to prepare for the computer[-based] ... Graph Round than it (was for) the [hand-drawn] 'charts' ... All in all, I consider [the system] a bonus [for] both the nurses and ... the patients ... providing the doctor ... doing the Graph Round is prepared to take more time to do it (Senior Register)

Clearly, the system offered the doctor a more effective system of surveillance but with an increased cost in terms of time. As we saw earlier, however, this did not translate itself in any greater efforts to control the activities of the patients; this was not a case of the 'carceral computer' (Lyon, 1988, p.99)

The computer system was also routinely used at the weekly clinics for dialysis patients held in the which was situated some distance away from the renal unit. In order to use the computer system a VDU terminal had to be taken on a trolley to the nurses' office in the department prior to the clinics. Rather strangely the major function of the computer system during these clinics was as a communication link with the renal unit. To ensure that the clinics had the most 'up to date' data on the patients a nurse would access the system and then copied it, by hand, onto the medical record for the doctors' reference. It was a cumbersome way to replace the telephone (the previous way the data was communicated)

The computer implementations compared: cui bono?

What emerges from a comparison of the two renal units is a paradox whereby the unit in which the consultants were most supportive of the system had the least support of the nursing staff while at the other unit the reverse was the case. The explanation of this lies, in important part, in the difference between the two units pre-existing manual systems of data collection and the relationship this had to the different styles of nursing organization.

At the Haemo Unit the nurses' work was explicitly patient-centred and had a relatively high sentimental work content which was applied to instil a high level of dialysis discipline among patients with the consequent higher level of emotional labour expected of the nurses than at the other unit. The introduction of the computer system involved these nurses in additional work with no obvious benefits for themselves. At the Dialysis Unit, by contrast, the nurses work explicitly focused on doctor-centred activities, in particular, providing the data and staff support for the clinics and medical meetings. Even though the nurses carried out sentimental work in their training of patients this aspect of their work was not appropriated by the doctors. In consequence, these nurses found the Renal Computer System saved themselves time and effort as well as providing a useful automated 'medical record summary' service to the junior doctors.

The two renal units were organized according to different principles. In the case of the Haemo Unit 'good patient care' was seen by the senior consultant as being as much about ensuring sound haemo-dialysis technique and diet as it was the practice of medicine. The priorities of the consultants at the Dialysis Unit were markedly different. Here the consultants did not recognise as part of their responsibility helping the patients to adjust to the discipline of renal dialysis. Instead, they emphasized the role of nephrology as a scientific enterprise. These different rationales were reflected in the organization and control of nursing work. The approach at the Haemo Unit was an inter-disciplinary and participatory as compared to the multi-disciplinary and hierarchical system at the Dialysis Unit.

Thc medical rationales are not, however, to be considered as wholly the outcomes of unfettered medical choice for the historical developments of the two renal units were important constraining influences. This was not the case at the Dialysis Unit where the renal unit and renal dialysis had developed as a necessary subsidiary to nephrology. The unit being bequeathed all the renal patients the nephrologists were unable to cure. It was because of these differences in rationales that the introduction and utilization of the computer system followed divergent paths at the two renal units and led to such paradoxical responses from the nursing and medical and of the system.

Conclusions

There have been a number of threads running through this chapter that interconnect with the theme that nurses have exhibited a marked tendency to be ambivalent about using computers. The tendency is not, however, a techno-phobic response rather it relates to the tendency for nurses to have to take on the responsibility for activities not carried out by others (Stacey, 1981). If a computer system is clearly perceived to benefit the nursing staff there is no evidence that they will reject it. This is clear from the renal clinical system where nurses welcomed the automation of the data collation they previously had carried out laboriously by hand and similarly, in the case of education and research including expert systems. The examination of both these areas (expert systems and clinical systems) has illuminated a key aspect of nursing that does characterise the general response to information technology. This is the sentimental work content to bedside care. Information technology whether developed for clinical purposes or resource management tends to ignore this and nurses themselves have not demonstrated any great degree of initiative ensuring systems also provide informational support for their work too. This, as Keen and Malby (1992) point out, is largely the consequence of a reluctance or inability to play organizational politics. Consequently, systems are implemented that provide clinical directors and business managers with information they can use while the nurses are left with the job of ensuring the systems are well fed with accurate data. Even the care planning systems have tended to develop into resource management systems rather than patient care systems for nurses.

7 Hospitals, IT and new organizational forms

Introduction

In all the previous chapters the character and dynamics of the social 'shaping' of healthcare computing and information technology have been central issues. In this chapter the focus is even less on the technological systems and more on the organizational arrangements within which they are embedded for there are currently a number of alternative theories which compete to explain the implications of our extensive reliance on computer systems within what has been termed 'information society' (Bell, 1980). The health service, for instance, is now an 'information rich' organization supported by a wide array of computer systems and this might lead one to believe that hospitals have become 'IT dependent' organizations (Rose, 1991) within this broader scenario. The debate around information society and its underlying post-industrial assumptions have been largely superseded by a newer set of discourses that share some of the assumptions of post-industrialism (Webster, 1995, p.218) and have come to take centre stage in the debate over the role and consequences of information and communications technologies in the near future.

The aim of this chapter is to relate these broader issues to current changes within hospital organization, IT and information systems. There are three main contenders to be considered: post-Fordism (including flexible specialisation) (Piore and Sabel, 1984), 'McDonaldization' (Ritzer, 1993) and postmodernism. Perhaps perversely (although it does provide a strong integrative focus), I am going to subordinate consideration of post-Fordism and 'McDonaldization' to the question whether or not postmodernism has any utility for the analysis of organizational change and putative IT-dependency within the NHS hospital sector. This approach will serve as an organizing principle for the analysis of the changing nature and role of hospital management (particularly the involvement of doctors as clinical directors) and governance. An important consideration will be that NHS hospitals are public sector organizations which, in contrast to the private sector, are managed according to conscious political choice. This gives rise to particular ideological and organizational contradictions as between state policy and local practice especially in relation to issues of managerial vs professional autonomy and control.

The chapter starts with a general discussion of postmodernism and organizational analysis (a necessary precursor to any consideration of hospital organization and management). There then follows a section on the recent organizational changes within the NHS hospital service and the ideological and organizational contradictions inherent within them. This leads into consideration as to how the restructuring might be best understood. It is here the issue of postmodernism is explored and done so in relation to 'McDonaldization' and post-Fordist interpretations of these changes. Having established my own position on the matter I then proceed to a specific hospital case study that has every appearance of being an exemplar of being a new form of organization. This is followed by a short conclusion.

Postmodernism and Organizations

Current debates surrounding postmodernism can be broadly summarised as being either in terms of *epistemology* or *periodization* (Cooper and Burrell, 1988; Parker, 1992; Hassard, 1993). In the terms adopted by Webster (1995, p.163) the first fascinates *postmodern thinkers* while the second relates to the putative *postmodern condition*. The two are not mutually exclusive although they tend to be clearly separated within the debates in the UK (e.g. Hassard and Parker, 1993).

(a) Epistemology: What is to be known?

Postmodernism is an assertion that the period of modernism has ended and that the Enlightenment project of emancipation based on human reason is at an end (Bauman, 1992). We can now see, so the argument runs, that there are limitations to human reason and it is therefore futile to pursue any such utopian scheme. If this is the case then organizational analysis is confronted with a major quandary as modern organizations are themselves products of human rationality. Weber's legal-rational bureaucracy was premised on the application of just such a notion even though it was not associated in Weber's mind with any emancipation or utopian project. If anything the reverse was the case for it was bureaucracy that provided the 'iron cage' of modern life and its 'disenchantment' (Albrow, 1970; Eldridge, 1973)

Postmodernism emerged out of the earlier post-structuralist discourse (Harvey 1989, p.41). Particularly significant is the work of Foucault especially his analysis of power/knowledge (Rabinow, 1984; Harvey, 1989, p.45). There is for Foucault an intimate link between systems of knowledge (discourse) and social control but only within particular localised contexts i.e. it is not possible to generalize. One major aspect of Foucault's work has been his extension of Bentham's model nineteenth century prison - the panopticon - in which inmates are continually under the surveillance of the central inspection tower whilst in their individual cells and controlled by a rigorous disciplinary code (Foucault, 1977). In the latter part of the twentieth century this model has been extended to modern organizations more generally but utilising computer technologies as the means of surveillance and control (Lyons, 1988, pp.97-9).

Control, however, is not the issue that the self-proclaimed post-modernists have been concerned with. They have been more pre-occupied with language. According to Lyotard (as an obvious example), all social activity is essentially a network of language games (Harvey, 1989, p.46). Within this framework organizational analysis becomes more a concern with 'the production of organization rather than the organization of production' (Cooper and Burrell, 1988, p.106). Moreover, it is futile to seek to construct any organizational meta-narrative but to concern ourselves with the inherent instability of organizations and their structures. It is more accurate from this perspective to view the organizations as the outcome of 'moves within a game' (rather than the outcome of overarching control systems/structures). Moreover, even the 'game' of analysis is driven by the contestability or 'agonistics' inherent in competitive games (Cooper and Burrell, 1988, p.98) and it is this alone that sets the limit to any organizational analysis. No grand theory is possible and the discourses will themselves be rooted in dissensus. Consensus means the end of the theoretical discourse (Cooper and Burrell, 1988, p.99). It is in this connection that Derridas contribution, according to Cooper (1989), is located for it is Derrida's contention that any assumption concerning the processes of rationality serves only to obscure the uncertainty that lies at the core of any social action (Cooper, 1989, pp.488-9). Instead one must identify the internal contradictions within these discourses by a process of de-construction (Derrida, 1978; 1981). The process of analysis being based on 'overturning the hierarchy at a given moment' and then stabilising the analysis by metaphorization (Derrida, 1981, p.41 quoted in Hassard, 1993, p.30).

The postmodern epistemology as applied to the sociology of organizations is less of a 'rupture' than some might claim. Phenomenology and the privileging of language and language games has long been an important strand in sociological and organizational thinking with much of the influence emanating from the work of Wittgenstein (Burrell and Morgan, 1979, pp.254-5). What is distinct about the current postmodern discourse, however, is the growing tendency to equate ontological uncertainty with organizational flexibility. Previously the concern had been with issues of 'efficiency' and 'effectiveness' (e.g. Albrow, 1970) and flexible - organic - forms more a management strategy of giving up control to keep control (Burns and Stalker, 1961; Fox, 1974). In practice, these remain major concerns of management. Now, so the argument seems to run, this involves the acceptance of new, more autonomous, organizational forms. It is to this issue of new organizational forms I now turn.

(b) Periodization: The postmodern epoch

At sometime in the 1980s there begun to be a realisation that the organizational forms that have dominated modern societies for the last 100 years were no longer appropriate, especially those characterised by hierarchy, centralized control systems and specialized division of labour (Reed, 1992, p.226). The newer, more flexible, forms of organization, categorized by Heydebrand (1989) as post-bureaucratic, where beginning to be recognised as not simply modifications but more thorough-going transformation from the pre-existing Fordist and bureaucratic forms to neo-/post-Fordist, flexible specialisation forms (Clegg, 1990; Reed, 1992). This transformation was a reflection of wider economic, social, and political as well as technological changes within society. For Heydebrand the emergence of post-bureaucratic forms 'are largely the result of the transition from industrial to post-industrial capitalism' (1989, p.323). The general view, however, has been less sanguine emphasizing more the result of an accommodation to the erosion of the West's privileged economic position and technological dominance *vis á vis* the rest of the world (e.g. Giddens, 1987, p.16; Harvey, 1989; 141-72; Webster, 1995, pp.140-7). The reality for Western economies has been one in which the post-war settlement based on Keynesian economics, Fordist production and consensus politics has increasingly failed (Jessop et al, 1988; Lash and Urry, 1987; Webster, 1995, pp.145-7).

The movement towards post-Fordist flexible specialisation (Piore and Sabel, 1984) and its variants reflect more the 'end of organized capitalism' (Lash and Urry, 1987), increasing globalization and the emergence of what Harvey (1989, p.147) has 'tentatively call[ed]' *flexible accumulation.* Within this new world order flexibility and innovation is crucial.

> It has entrained rapid shifts in the patterning of uneven development ... It has also entailed a new round of ... 'time-space compression' ... the time horizons of private and public decision-making have shrunk, while satellite communication and declining transport costs have made it increasingly possible to spread those decisions immediately over an ever wider and variegated space. (Harvey, 1989, p.147)

According to this version of postmodernity, *productionist* values no longer dominate the economic and political agendas and in their place *consumerist* ones are now in ascendance. A view that has some correspondence with Baudrillard's version of the shift from modern to post-modern society and with it the imperatives of production has been replaced by a new system of images and signs in which the distinction between the real and its representations is problematic (Baudrillard, 1983; Smart, 1992, pp.123- 7). For Baudrillard (1983, p.154 n.4), following McLuhhan, views the 'medium as the message' i.e. there has occurred an implosion of 'the medium' and 'the real' giving rise to a nebulous hyperreality that erases their differences and distinctiveness (Smart, 1992, p.127). This 'implosion' plays a crucial role in the mobilization of consumers and the creation of a new social order in which consumer power is more crucial than labour power within cybernetic capitalism (Baudrillard, 1975, p.144 cited in Smart 1992, p.121). The only certainty, it seems, is the uncertainty of the (world) markets within which changing patterns of consumption are closely related both to the growing ascendancy of post-modern tastes and ideas (Lash, 1990; Featherstone, 1991). This 'specialized consumption' (Lash 1990, pp.39-40) is reflected in the growth of niche markets (Clegg, 1990, p.181).

For Lash (1990) the change in consumption 'is in all likelihood cultural' (Lash 1990, p.41) and marked by a shift from *differentiation* to *de-differentiation*. The latter term having a certain amount in common with the work of Baudrillard (Lash 1990, p.5). The modernist tendency was towards *differentiation* (Lash 1990 11-12). Thus the archetypal modernist organization was the Weberian legal-rational model characterised by hierarchy and functional specialisation. This is now being replaced, so the argument runs, by a post-modernist version in which modular, multi/inter-disciplinary teams replace functional hierarchies; a process of *de-differentiation*. We can see this also occurring in the case of technology. With the introduction of digital technology, for instance, it is now possible to integrate previously functional distinct technologies e.g. telephones, faxes, computers and CDs and thereby de-differentiating between image, sound/music and text. The post-Fordist organization (whether or not it is postmodern) can be assumed to be highly dependent upon information and communications technology (ICT) which may, according to Heydebrand (1989, p.342), '[open] the door to flexible and informal social arrangements in the workplace and to a post-hierarchical form of organization'.

I now to turn to the case of the NHS (more precisely, the hospital service) for it strikes me as a particularly 'interesting case'. It has become a 'workbench' for new organizational forms designed to change health care delivery from a professionally (*producer*) defined service to a patient (*consumer*) defined marketplace. At least, that was the official rhetoric of the 1989 White Paper *Working for Patients*. The subsequent NHS and Community Care Act, 1990, was intended to transform health authorities into 'champions of the people' with a duty to consult consumer interests closely (Ranade, 1994, p.71). These changes may, however, be less a commitment to consumerism than a simulacram designed for other more modernist purposes such as 'efficiency' and 'effectiveness'. It is to this general question I now turn.

The UK Health Service as a modernist project

The NHS, according to the Labour politician, writer and journalist Michael Foot, was 'the greatest Socialist achievement of the [post-war] Labour government' (Foot, 1973).

> It was the first health system in any Western Society to offer free medical care to the entire population. It was, furthermore, the first comprehensive system to be based not on the insurance principle ... but on the national provision of services available to everyone ... (Klein, 1989, p.1)

It has become the exemplar of what the modernist project could achieve. The organizational structure designed to deliver this service was highly bureaucratic and apparently based on the modernist principle of rationality. At the same time there existed another principle that appeared to contradict it that of professional autonomy. In the hands of the doctors professional autonomy had become translated into a medical dominance (Freidson, 1970) within the hospitals which had always enabled them to avoid policies they - as a group - did not agree with (Dent 1995a). This in itself did not undermine the modernist logic of the service for while professional autonomy injects an ambiguity into bureaucracy it has, nevertheless, been there since Weber (e.g. Albrow, 1970) and on closer examination will be found to be in more of a symbiotic relation than first appears to be the case.

The NHS is a particularly good example of a modernist project one designed to free the people from the burden of illness and disease. But medical dominance (Freidson, 1970) put substantial organizational and financial strains of the NHS. This is not a situation unique to the UK and similar conditions exist in Europe and the USA. For example, see The Milbank Quarterly's volume on 'The Changing Character of the Medical Profession' (1988), Freddi and Björkman's (1989) edited volume on 'health governance' and more recently Johnson, Larkin and Saks' *Health Professions and the State in Europe* (1994). The evidence points to all Western governments trying to reduce the autonomy of doctors as a method of containing the cost of health care services. This has concentrated the attention of many analysts on the concept and issue of medical autonomy and the prospects of deprofessionalization and/or proletarianization of doctors.

Within the NHS many hospital consultants have been incorporated within the new organizational arrangements as clinical directors and thereby avoiding erosion of their status whilst at the same time changing their professional role within the hospital division of labour (see Dent, 1993). This development has been closely related to the growing centrality of (quasi-) market relations and the commodification of health services. This is the obverse side to the same 'coin' as the putative 'deprofessionalization' of doctors. Whether this coinage is postmodern or of 'high', or 'late' modernism (Giddens, 1990) cannot be answered yet for it is first necessary to identify in more detail what changes actually have taken place in the organization of the NHS hospital service.

From hierarchies to markets

The immediate rationality for introducing market mechanisms into the NHS had been essentially to control its escalating costs (Ham et al, 1990, pp.11-20; Ham, 1992, pp.38-59) and, in the process, eroding the long-standing dominance of the NHS biggest spenders, the doctors. In the process the changes have begun to erode the general principle of universal provision according to 'procedural rules' to a pragmatic one of 'getting things done'. A characteristic Heydebrand (1989, pp.343) identifies with new (non-bureaucratic) organizational forms. Gone are the rational principles of planning and priorities within an integrated service. In their place there now exists the imperative of 'consumer' demand (the inverted commas are essential here) in an internal market of competing hospitals, clinics and general practice, etc. The movement towards marketization, however, has not been in any sense a unilinear one and the general strategy of the British Conservative administration has been more heterogenous than might be implied from the summary so far. This can be clearly shown with reference to the three major policy innovations much referred to throughout earlier chapters:

1. The *Griffith's Inquiry* (1983) recommended a single line of management supported by effective management information systems (Scrivens 1988) to replace the consensus management introduced the previous decade.

2. The introduction of the *Resource Management Initiative*(DHSS, 1986) with the conscious management of meanings and symbols (culture) to bring about the incorporation of medicine into management with doctors accepting the need for financial constraints on their clinical activities

3 The White Paper *Working for Patients* (Secretary of State for Health and Others, 1989) furthered this process with proposals for a new management system that integrated financial and quality controls to deliver 'a good, cost effective, service' to patients (para. 1.13). It was not, however, until the subsequent legislation - *NHS and Community Act of 1990* - that (quasi-) market principles were overtly injected into this new decentralized model of the health service in the UK.

Even so the policy was not as overtly market oriented as Margaret Thatcher, the then prime minister, had wanted for she, apparently, had wanted the actual privatization of hospitals and clinics and the encouragement of private health insurance (Marmor and Plowden, 1991, p.17). Instead, what emerged was the concept of the 'internal market' which has many parallels with the US concept of Health Maintenance Organizations (HMO) as outlined by Enthoven (1985). In this new system the health authorities are responsible for identifying the health needs of the community and *purchasing* (i.e. acting as a consumer) from hospitals and clinics, etc. who are the *providers* (producers) of the services. The General Practitioners are also intended to become *purchasers* (consumers) on behalf of their patients within this 'marketplace'. This new system is based on a separation of functions between the *purchaser* and the provider of health services. The purchaser has the duty to obtain the 'best' price and quality service for the patients. It does this through 'contracting out' to different hospitals which are (formally at least) in competition with each other. Many of these hospitals are now 'self-governing' trusts operating, in principle, as independent commercial enterprises within the internal market.

Accounting for treatment

In order to meet the requirements of the internal market and particularly the new contractual arrangements all hospitals are now required to install comprehensive resource management and quality assurance information/IT systems (Packwood et al., 1991; Dent, 1993; Keen, 1994). resource management (RM), has been defined by its Directorate (Bullas, 1989, para. 1.2) as 'a hospital management process involving doctors, nurses and other clinical and managerial staff in strategic and operational decision making ... a process underpinned by a patient based information system'. The supporting information system, known as the 'case-mix management' is intended to provide the means of costing treatment and hospital care at the level of the patient and is based closely on the DRG system used in US but referred to instead as 'Health Related Groups' (HRGs). (see p. 53 for details).

As already mentioned it is the government's clear policy intention that hospital doctors will become fully incorporated within the NHS (rather than the accommodation that could be said to describe the pre-existing situation) and to this end the resource management arrangements are designed to make hospital consultants directly responsible for their clinic budgets. The success of the new arrangements, however, remains unproven and the limited evidence that does exist is far from promising. The resource management project was implemented experimentally at six hospitals and the results, particularly in connection with the IT, can only be described as mixed for, as Packwood et al. (1991, p.44) reported:

> [T]he [hospitals] ... found that ... implementing systems ... took much longer than originally imagined. ... the[y] had to learn as they went. [Hospitals] also reported that they lacked sufficient NHS staff to cope with such a large-scale implementation. Taken together, this meant that often the flow of data ... got worse before it got better.

The coding and patient classification systems that lay at the heart of the case mix system were not used routinely at any of the hospitals (with the partial exception of one). Packwood et al. (ibid., p.50) commented that 'involvement was patchy, and most work in this area remained experimental', whilst, the state of the nursing systems was even worse, reflecting 'patchy developments at all sites ... [and] little to show for a great deal of effort' (ibid., p.53). From the evidence of this study it was clear that the NHS can not rely on IT to provide a 'technological fix', at least, not in the short term. Although that does not preclude it having an important role to play in providing support for the new information/organizational systems once the nurses, doctors and managers are fully familiar with the new systems and know what they want of the IT.

The programme of changes in the NHS has been in process for some time (certainly since the Griffith's Inquiry in 1983). The transformation has been from an hierarchical, centrally funded, administrative system with a division of labour dominated by the medical profession to a *formally* decentralized system of autonomous hospitals, etc. in (quasi-) market competition with each other. These new arrangements are intended to be managed within hospitals by inter-disciplinary teams of business managers and health care professionals headed by senior doctors in the role of clinical directors. These arrangements are intended to reflect a new patient-centred service that is beginning to be co-ordinated and integrated via a complex IT-based system. Having clarified what constitutes the new arrangements and information systems it is now possible to assess whether the changes correspond to some notion of postmodernity and whether such a notion has meaning.

Changes in the National Health Service: Hospitals and 'burger restaurants

The UK government has overseen the introduction of the following measures that can be seen as post-bureaucratic (Heydebrand, 1989). Whether these can also be taken as indicating a postmodern turn in the organization of hospitals requires greater scrutiny:

1. The commodification of health service provision with the introduction of detailed cost and quality controls (Tuckman and Blackburn, 1991; Starkey, 1992).

2. Transforming the relation between patient and hospital from 'supplicant' to 'consumer' and thereby changing health care provision from being a citizens' right to a being simply a customer service (Cox, 1992, pp.34-8; Ranade, 1994, pp.65-8).

3. Comprehensive IT systems to underpin the new management information systems and facilitate the organizational changes (See Chapter 3).

To achieve these objectives the state administration has pursued a strategy of actively transmuting the NHS culture (Ranade, 1994, pp.82-99) from one dominated by professionalism and 'rational paternalism' (Klein, 1989) to one imbued with the rhetoric of the market.

The NHS currently comprises a great many hospital trusts which are organizationally autonomous contractors to the health authorities. The health workers (including the professions) are being re-organized into polyvalent groupings (or the work has been 'contracted out') while the whole health care system is being underpinned by increasingly sophisticated IT systems. This new and still emergent version of the NHS has much in common with the new and postmodern organizational forms identified by Heydebrand (1989) and Clegg, (1990). The new NHS system could even be said to have much in common with a system of franchising very similar to Benetton's (Clegg 1990, pp.120-5) with the hospitals franchised by the Department of Health to 'sell' health care services so long as they comply with detailed quality standards. Again, like Benetton, these NHS hospitals are supposed to have IT systems that provide itemized details, including costs, of each patient's treatment and 'hotel-type' services (although in practice the system aims at average and not actual individual costs based on HRGs - see Chapter 3).

To label an organizational arrangement as 'postmodern' because it corresponded with the dimensions on Clegg's model (1990, p.203) would, however, be over-simplistic. It is equally possible to recast the franchise model as a variant of Weber's legal-rational bureaucratic organization. The alternative here is Ritzer's (1993) 'McDonaldization' thesis which argues that the pressures to control costs and increase efficiency has given rise (in the US) to a new form of bureaucratic control within hospitals akin to those of a fast food restaurant (1993, pp.52-5, 79-80, 139-41). There are, according to Ritzer, four basic dimensions at the heart of the McDonald's model (1993, p.9). First, *efficiency*, based on Taylorist and Fordist principles of work organization. Second, a service that can be *quantified and calculated* both in terms of how the tasks are performed and in the price and quality of the product. Thirdly, *predictability*, so that no matter in which McDonald's restaurant you eat you always eat exactly the same food. Finally, *control* by replacing human skills and knowledge with technology. What is distinct about this system of control is that it is not exercised through a monolithic corporate hierarchy but through a tightly controlled franchising arrangement. There is a prima facie case that the internal market within the NHS works in a similar way. The new franchised' arrangements between hospitals and health authorities and general practitioners (i.e. purchaser-provider relations) have led to a 'McDonaldization' (Ritzer, 1993) of the system. The extreme rationalization of hamburger-style franchised and standardized catering is possible, however, because it does not require the presence of expertise on site. This is not the case with either cordon bleu restaurants or NHS acute hospitals. In the case of hospitals, these continue to remain dependent upon the professional expertise and autonomy of the doctors rather than standardized pricing systems and quality controls. In Ritzer's (1993, p.141) own view, '[t]he ultimate irrationality of the rationalization of medicine would be the unanticipated consequences of a decline in the quality of medical practice and a deterioration in the health of the patients'. For this reason he asserts that 'health professions and their patients need to learn how to control rational structures and institutions to ameliorate their irrational consequences' (1993, p.141).

Whilst one can identify elements of 'McDonaldization' within the new internal market arrangements, particularly, the franchise-type relations between health authorities and hospitals there are also important differences. Firstly, the central role of professional expertise limits the extent to which new technologies can replace the doctor. There remains an important role for judgement and discretion in the management and treatment of ill health. Secondly, measurement and assessment of the quality of service is not limited to the patients' or managers' evaluations. Medical staff, unlike staff working at a McDonald's restaurant, will claim an ascendancy in judging whether their work is of a high quality or not. Thirdly, the organization of hospitals is not determined by the quasi-franchiser (i.e. the health authority) it is for the staff and management at the individual hospitals to decide. There is, in short, more flexibility than is available to a McDonald's franchisee. Far more problematic for a postmodern interpretation is the post-Fordist organizational model.

Postmodernism vs post-Fordism

The new organizational forms identified as postmodern by Clegg, (1990) are more frequently categorized as post-Fordist (Reed, 1992, p.230). Very few analysts, other than Clegg (1990), Reed (1992, pp.226- 37) and Boje and Dennehy (1993) have been prepared to conflate the two models (postmodernism and post-Fordism). There are important distinctions to be made between the two models (not least the different emphases put on cultural and economic influences on organizational forms) which makes it unwise for the two to be fused together. Nevertheless, it may still be the case that they are cognately closely interconnected. It is this possibility (and its implications) that is to be explored here.

The new organizational arrangements within the NHS are the consequence of a politically driven post-Fordism of a right-wing kind (to paraphrase Rustin, 1989, p.75) and despite much government rhetoric the search has been for new forms of organizational control rather than finding new and more flexible ways of providing consumer choice. Nevertheless, in searching for new solutions that met their own criteria the Conservative administration opened up the multiplicity of power relations (dominated by the medical profession) that characterises hospitals. It is within this space of 'unintended consequences' that we find elements of postmodernity beginning to permeate the public sector of health care in the UK. In order to develop this point it is necessary to return to the distinction was made earlier as between the epistemology and periodization of postmodernism. The epistemology component pointed to a widespread loss of faith in rationalist discourses such as scientific management and contingency theory. A consequence has been that management discourse has become vulnerable to the 'agonistics' of postmodern language games and Derridean deconstruction. This interpretation does not, however, offer a basis for claiming that the introduction of the (managed) market meant that NHS hospitals have become postmodern. Such an assertion would need to rely on Lash's (1990) and Lash and Urry's (1994) argument relating to concepts of *de-differentiation* and *aestheticization*. Just as digitalization has fundamentally changed the relationship between computers, compact discs, videos and communication technologies (Lash, 1990, p.12) so too have management techniques and strategies changed with the shift from predominantly bureaucratic to market-oriented organizational forms. This general shift has been underpinned by the adoption of proselytising management cultures which reflect - to borrow a term favoured by Lash (1990) and Lash and Urry (1994) - an increasing aestheticization of management. We also find the social nature of health and ill health has also undergone important changes. They have, to a large extent, been transformed from medically (i.e. producer) defined conditions à la Talcott Parsons (e.g. Gerhardt, 1987) to becoming consumer goods. This is something for which the UK government is not solely responsible, witness the popular interest in jogging, aerobics and health maintenance activities (and the related goods and services on offer in the private sector). Nevertheless, in attempting to displace the centrality of allopathic medicine by preventive methods of health promotion the administration has placed greater weight on the citizens' interpretation of their own health needs and demands. There is, in short, a growing aestheticization of health. This, according to Lash and Urry (1994), would be a sign of postmodernism although they overlook the point in their own analysis of the NHS.

Lash and Urry (1994, p.15) claim a distinction can be made between cognitive and aesthetic goods:

> What is increasingly being produced [in contemporary political economies] are not material objects, but signs. These signs are primarily of two types. Either they have a primarily cognitive content and thus are post-industrial or informational goods. Or they primarily have an aesthetic, *in the broadest sense of the aesthetic*, content and are primarily postmodern goods ... ' (*emphases added*)

This distinction is derived from Baudrillard's notion of 'sign value' which is counter-posed to the modernist (Marxist) concept of 'exchange value' and pre-modernist 'use-value' and is a particularly abstract concept, a 'simulacrum of a simulacrum'. The aestheticization of goods takes place through the design process and 'branding' by which marketers and advertisers attach images to goods. It also occurs through the complicity of producers and consumers in, for instance, the semiotic work carried out by tourists on their travels (Urry, 1990) and, by extension, patients undergoing treatment. The distinction between cognitive and aesthetic signs offers an interesting and possibly useful way of beginning to analyze the new organizational forms emerging within the NHS. This is not a view, however, shared by Lash and Urry (1994, p.210) themselves. They argue that whilst the changes that have taken place are of a post-Fordist kind they have not led to a post-Fordist (let alone postmodernist) transformation. There are three reasons, they tell us, for this being the case:

1. It is not clear who are the consumers and therefore to whom the managers need to respond most directly;

2. The information and contracting structures underpinning the quasi-market arrangements requires more, not less, bureaucratic hierarchies;

3. The work of doctors has become more Fordist with the introduction of the new contracts and medical audit following the 1989 White Paper.

These points, however, misinterpret the impact of the changes. Firstly, the issue of who are the consumers? Currently, the health authorities and fundholding general practitioners are the purchasers on behalf of the patient/consumers of the services. The health authorities, however, are obliged to monitor closely their citizenry's' views and experience of the health services (e.g. Ranade, 1994, pp.110-12). This corresponds with private sector management carrying out market surveys and the like.

Secondly, to counter the allegation that the internal market requires more, not less, bureaucracy. It is true that between 1989 and 1991 there was nearly a threefold increase of managers in the NHS (Ranade, 1994, p.73). This reflected a move from an administered to a managed system in which the government devolved increasing responsibilities to the hospital managers with the intention of constituting them as a countervailing power to doctors (Robinson, 1994, p.6). The growth was part of the general 'histrionics' of the new managerialism and intended to ensure eventual acceptance of the new organizational order (Cox, 1991, p.99). Neither of these points add up to a growth in bureaucracy even if it has meant more managers.

Finally, the assumption that contracting and medical audit means a more Fordist work situation' for doctors. As I have argued elsewhere (Dent, 1993, p.267) the reality has been more of incorporation than subordination (or deprofessionalization or proletarianization). Previously, the arrangements between the NHS and the medical profession might best be described as one of accommodation. With the introduction of new contracts and medical audit, however, expectations on the part of managers and doctors have certainly changed. Nevertheless, it remains the case that it is the doctors themselves who determine the criteria defining the quality of medical care.

In general terms the argument I am pursuing here is that hospitals have taken on a predominantly post-Fordist organizational form as a direct consequence of government policy. In the process, however, they have undergone further changes corresponding with Lash (1990) and Lash and Urry's (1994) notions of *de-differentiation* and *aestheticization* in the organization and delivery of health care services. It is these that are the postmodern elements within the new organizational arrangements. In order to avoid any over-generalizations and to illustrate what I have in mind I will now turn to a case study of a specific general hospital.

The new hospital case study: A soft organizational approach

The hospital was a new and relatively small general hospital which employed 35 full-time consultants the vast majority of whom had only been recently appointed. The nursing staff equated to 400 (i.e. Whole Time Equivalents). At the time of the study it was less than ten years old and had another year to go before it became a Trust and so too had the General Manager before his title would change to 'Chief Executive Officer'. 'New Hospital' is not its real name but adopted to ensure the anonymity of those interviewed. The hospital is located in an ever growing 'new town' which is the industrial centre of an otherwise rural part of the country. The case study was carried out over the period 1991 to 1993 with most interviews being carried out over the period September to April, 1992-93. Data was collected from semi-structured taped interviews with informants drawn from management, doctors and nurses (i.e. directly involved in the management processes).

The soft organizational form

At 'New Hospital' the General Manager implemented his chosen interpretation of the edicts of the resource management and the *NHS and Community Care Act* (1990) in a peculiarly participative way. It was a culturalist policy decided on by himself but implemented participatively. This *aestheticization* process can be viewed as an organizational equivalent of *populist ventriloquism* given that the General Manager was introducing his preferred system in the name of participation and involvement (Hall et al., 1978 cited in Jessop et al., 1988, pp.71- 2). The General Manager defined this strategy as his 'soft organizations' approach. 'I want to do a bit of business, I want to see people, ... I ... mak[e] connections - ... what you would call 'soft' organizational communications - [these] are extremely easy around here ...'. The idea is analogous to the postmodern architecture of Krier who has rejected sky-scrapers and tower blocks in favour of more small local communities 'cities within cities' (cited in Harvey, 1989, pp.67-8). Neither the architect nor the manager is being nostalgic for a romanticised pre-modern past but is seeking alternatives to modernist arrangements. In the case of the hospital it is an attempt by the General Manager to carve out a niche within the National Health Service that Peters and Waterman (1982) would describe as 'skunk works':

> [A part of an organization characterised by an] almost radical *decentralization* and *autonomy*, with its attendant *overlap, messiness* around the edges, *lack of co-ordination*, internal competition, and somewhat *chaotic* conditions, in order to breed the entrepreneurial spirit' (cited in Ritzer, 1993, pp.180-1, *emphases* in the original).

Within this niche the General Manager's own strategy seemed to share some commonality with the proponents of Soft Systems Methodology (SSM) (Checkland 1981; Checkland and Scholes, 1991). Moreover, the proponents of SSM even suggest (apparently without irony) that their approach may be postmodern:

> [SSM can be] used not so much to plan calculative action ... but rather to guide and make sense of the discourse [of re-organization]. This is, perhaps, *postmodern* .... SSM is being used to help an observer community which constructs interpretations of the world, these *interpretations* having no universal status. New interpretations have led to new ways of structuring and managing [organizations] but not in any absolute or Utopian sense ... (Checkland and Scholes, 1990, pp.235-6 *some emphases added*).

Similarly, within the hospital the General Manager acted as a 'guide' and 'interpreter'. Thus, the 'soft' organizational arrangements were consciously not constructed to alienate the doctors but to incorporate them into a central role within the new organizational arrangements. Instead of adopting the officially recommended clinical directorate model a different inter-disciplinary model was adopted (see Figure 7.1). This was one based on the clinical units (e.g. General Medicine, Surgery, Paediatrics, etc.). Each chaired by a consultant who was also, automatically, a member of the Hospital Management Board. The doctors, consequently, were (numerically) more strongly represented they would have been under a Clinical Directorate system. At the same time the 'board' was a large and an unwieldy body and functioned primarily to formalise decisions agreed on a day-to-day informal basis. Each clinical unit was headed by a consultant doctor and supported by a senior nurse. The work of these inter-disciplinary teams was co-ordinated by one of two associates General Managers both of whom were nurses. This arrangement was to ensure that the work of the different units co-ordinated overall as well as giving the nurses, as a body, power and influence within the new structure.

The centrality of the consultants to the 'soft organizational system' was further reinforced by their being accommodated in offices near to the General Manager (and certainly nearer than those of the managers). This provided the consultants with easy access to the General Manager but it also ensured he would have privileged access to the medics own informal networks:

> I've moved all the consultants so that they are all on this floor, here.... Purely, because the view is that those 'lads' [*sic*] are the ones that are going to 'screw you up'. They have several needs. One of their needs is to be near me - and loved by me! ... And I've got a need to see the 'whites of their eyes' so I know what's worrying them. So, on the *informal* network ... you 'smell' the ... 'smoke' on the Monday morning and by doing that you can feed back through the *informal* network very quickly. (General Manager)

At the same time the doctors previous 'power-base' in the organizational structure, the Medical Executive Committee (pre-existing in all NHS hospitals) was replaced by the Unit Medical Advisory Committee with no formal powers itself.

The consultants, however, were not naively seduced by the model. As one consultant surgeon explained, 'our view ... was [that] ... either we were going to be managed by managers (who in many cases have no idea what they're doing) or we would ... manage ourselves'. Nevertheless, these same consultants did not find the official Clinical Directorate model particularly appealing because of the greater demand on their time it was believed to involve. This lack of popularity for the official model was shared by doctors at a nearby hospital too where clinical directorates had been introduced. It emerged from an interview with a clinical director that the General Manager had needed to cajole consultants into taking on this new role and that his colleagues had decided that he would be the best person for the job because 'they didn't want it ... [and] I am by far the youngest' (Clinical Director). The general policy at this other hospital had been to implement the new organizational arrangements contained in the *NHS and Community Care Act* (1990) as if they were bureaucratic edicts which contrasted markedly with the 'soft' organizational approach of the 'New Hospital'. The approach here was more flexible, informal and far more effective at actively involving the doctors in the management of the hospital. An example of this was the General Manager's strategy relating to the issue of 'Trust' status (i.e. the hospital to become organizationally autonomous within the NHS). As one of the consultants explained:

> [When] the hospital opened ... I think there w[as] a general, almost unanimous, viewpoint among the consultants that they didn't want anything to do with [Trust status] .... Over the next year [however] ... it really gathered momentum .... I'm not sure we ever made any conscious decision ... It just [be]came clear that the majority of people of people wanted to go that way.

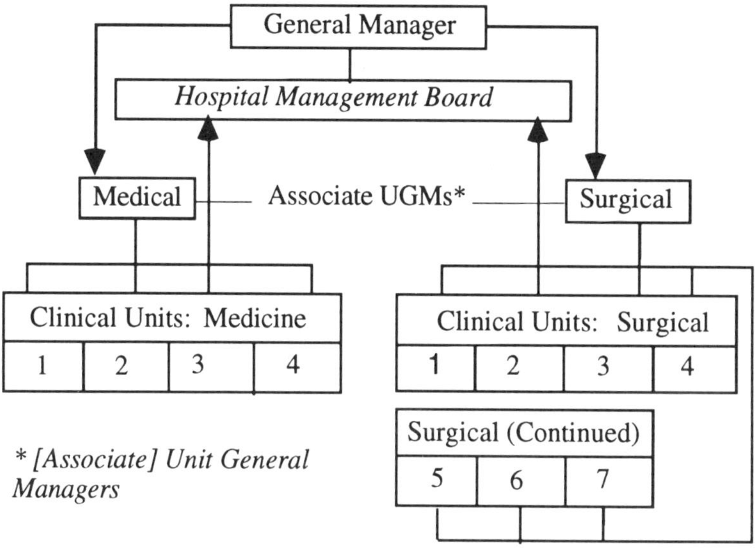

Figure 7.1 Organizational chart of the New Hospital (simplified)

An example of the aesthetics of a proselytizing manager utilizing a *populist ventriloquist* strategy (Hall et al., 1978 cited in essop et al., 1988, pp.71-2). The consultants were not prepared to see 'Trust' status, having any direct impact on their work situation even though they accepted the reality of budgetary constraints. An acceptance generally shared by UK doctors. According to Harrison and Schulz (1989, p.203), they now regard, 'overall financial limitations as being legitimate restrictions on their autonomy ... '. They, nevertheless, would be hostile to any external controls on their clinical practice. As one paediatrician put the point: 'We don't anticipate [Trust status] changing our work patterns one iota because if it does there will be 'holy hell' to pay and the ... General Manager knows that.'. Nevertheless, within the three years of opening the medical staff had accepted shared responsibility for managing the delivery of the clinical services within budgetary constraints.

Whilst the management at the 'New Hospital' adopted a flexible organizational response to the new internal market it cannot be said that there was really any adequate IT to support the new arrangements of the kind assumed by the proponents of post-bureaucratic organizations whether of a post-Fordist or post-modern kind (Heydebrand, 1989; Clegg, 1990). A situation that was largely the consequence of the limitations on the resources and services provided by the health authority.

The hospital was provided with an extensive set of IT systems covering the core patient-related activities, staffing and finances as well as more specialist laboratory systems and the like. These systems, however, were wholly inadequate for the demands of resource management. This was a matter of some concern to those working at the hospital but was certainly not a unique situation for it was compatible with the research findings from the NHS resource management experimental sites cited earlier (Packwood et al., 1991, p.44).

It was the responsibility of the resource management (RM) project team to provide the IT policy and advice internal to the 'New Hospital'. Yet none of the members of the RM Project Team were particularly knowledgeable about computing or IT generally having followed careers in NHS administration or nursing previously. In an attempt to overcome this problem the RM Project Manager was assisted by the computing specialists employed by the health authority. The computer systems already in place were, in any case, provided by the health authority although it was generally agreed that these systems were limited in the services they could provide being, as they were, based on rather antiquated ICL) systems. The General Manager at the 'New Hospital' took a pragmatically fatalistic view on the situation viewing the health authority's systems and service as the most cost effective they were likely to get. As he explained, 'instinctively I would have them *decentralized* but practically I think we've got to be *centralized* because of the "economies of scale" ...' (*emphases added*). The view of the health authority directorate was that they too believed they had a role to play in the area of hospital computing services '[we are taking] the view ... [that] resource management ... was about [hospital] 'ownership' *but* with [a] .. central steer and policy direction [from us] mainly on issues of IT' (Director of Purchasing and Quality Assurance [QA]).

In practice, both the health authority and the hospital had inherited expensive systems from the regional authority which when coupled with the vested interests of the computer specialists seriously hindered the introduction of more flexible IT systems more appropriate to the hospital's new requirements.

As time passed and the ramifications of the new purchaser-provider relations became clearer the health authority's 'central steer' could be seen to be operating not in the area of IT but primarily over issues of 'quality assurance' and 'medical audit'. This was because quality issues were mandatory elements within the new 'internal market' arrangements whereas IT was not.

To start with the quality measures in relation to medical work were very general:

> You will not have people sitting in Outpatients' for three hours. You ... will tell GPs that someone has been discharged within 24 hours. ... [T]hese are the very practical things we are saying to ... [the hospitals] ... and that's been helpful because its actually structured the debate - made quality much more tangible. (Director of Purchasing and QA)

In the longer term, however, the purchasing health authority would become increasingly interested in the results of medical audit 'in a management sense' and these would be 'picked up through the contracting process ... in [asking] "OK, what's your re-admission rate like? What's your operation failures like?" Those sorts of things we will be writing into contracts' (Director of Purchasing and QA). Medical audit was one area in which the hospital did have its own IT support and which was separate from the rest of the hospital. This was to ensure confidentiality and protect medical autonomy whilst the doctors attempted to develop adequate systems of medical audit (see Chapter 5).

None of the systems within the New Hospital', however, were in any way sophisticated enough to be part of a fully integrated new organizational form as anticipated by Heydebrand (1989). If anything, the technology hampered the emergence locally of new organizational arrangements that combined a post-Fordist strategy (of incorporating medical staff) with a post-modern *de-differentiation* and *aestheticization* within the organizational culture.

NHS hospitals and postmodernity: Tentative conclusions

Consideration of postmodern elements has enabled the analysis to be extended beyond the limitations of the productionist focus of post-Fordism and the modernist interpretations of Lash and Urry (1994). For unless we take into account the newly negotiated cultures and aesthetics of the hospitals' new organizational forms our understanding of the impact of these changes will be limited. It is the intertwining between the post-Fordist flexibilities and postmodern cultural aestheticization that gives rise to the range of de-differentiated organizational forms within the service. These reflect local circumstances, resources and possibilities both within the community and the organization (most patients will be citizens living within the local community). The loose-coupling and budgetary constraints of the 'internal market' have not given rise to any significant 'McDonaldization' of the NHS as the commodification of ill health has begun to take hold. This is largely related to the continued role being played by medical dominance and professionalism that, whilst changed in some important respects, remains. A point to be returned to in the next and concluding chapter. Instead of a process of deprofessionalization, doctors have suffered nothing worse than a comfortable incorporation within the new system as senior managers.

The inclusion of the case study was an attempt to explicate the way in which the aestheticization of management and the de-differentiation of the organization may be realised locally. Further, it was intended to elucidate why local management practices and organizational arrangements are not to be understood as epiphenomena or residual categories but as an essential component to any analysis. Thus, the 'soft organization' model was the metaphor that made sense of the organizational arrangements and management strategies within the hospital. The underlying imagery paralleled that claimed for Checkland's Soft Systems Methodology in that it was a localised interpretation as to how the hospital's organization was to be constructed and managed. It enabled the General Manager to orchestrate a flexible, informally networked and autonomous, organization. This was a serious game in which the organizational players recognise very clearly the inherent instability of the 'internal market' and the implications this could have for their relations with other players within the NHS. In this context, the 'soft organizational' form was neither wholly pragmatic nor simply a deceptive gloss for a 'McDonaldized' standardized franchise. Firstly, the signification of the organizational form was one that has been assigned to it through a process of aestheticization rather than technical rationality (i.e. it was the legitimation of the informal networks over the formal management structures that characterised this organizational form). Secondly, the health authorities were unable to impose any contractual requirements that would equate to McDonaldization. Nor was the 'New Hospital' management (including senior medical and nurse personnel) seeking to respond to the imperatives of the internal market in a way commensurable with that highly rationalized form. Instead they were intent on adapting and developing their own autonomy and flexibility in a manner more in line with post-bureaucratic (Heydebrand, 1989, p.327) or a postmodern organizational form (Clegg, 1990, p.181). It was an organization in which the culture was politically used to integrate an otherwise loosely coupled, centrifugal system of complex and fragmentary relational forms - to 'hybridize' the words of Heydebrand (1989) and Clegg (1990). Lyotard's assertion that the postmodern discourse is driven by 'agonistics' may be relevant in terms of theorization/epistemology but the consequences of the new organizational forms are more real than just a competitive interest in discourse. It is associated with a process Lash and Urry (1987) have referred to as the disorganization of capital and represents a new order akin to 'high technology feudalism'. It is an organizational world in which 'legal rationality' has only localised significance. 'The opposition to "reason" frequently attributed to "postmodern" analyses is, to be more precise ... an opposition to a totalizing idea of reason ... There is no "postmodern" opposition to rationality *per se*. Rather it is the existence of a plurality of "rationalities"'(Smart, 1992, p.180). In these terms it is perfectly possible that the postmodern, post-bureaucratic, organization may imply a dystopian and disorganized future within late capitalism (e.g. Lash and Urry, 1994, p.12), an interpretation that may well apply to the NHS hospital service.

8 Professions, IT and Hospital Management

Introduction

In this final chapter I will attempt to meld together the various accounts and arguments presented in the different chapters. I will start with a section on the professions which contrasts their role in the governance of hospitals with to their potential proletarianization within information society. Next comes a final excursion into the realms of healthcare computing. This section is partly aimed at addressing the question of how to avoid being dated and irrelevant even before publication given the rapid developments in computer technologies? In dealing with that issue I also take the opportunity to describe and comment on some current key developments, including document imaging processing (DIP) and clinical workstations, which are being currently introduced but have not until now been discussed within this book. This will lead into a revisitation of the social constructionist argument and the work of computer specialists, doctors and nurses. There then follows the final section on the emergence of a professional-managerial cadre in NHS hospitals and the ambiguous role played by computer-based health information systems.

Professions and governance

Hospital computing and IT, along with information and communications technologies (ICTs), present us with two competing scenarios in terms of their implications for professional occupations: the 'optimistic' and the 'pessimistic'. The first is the post-industrialisation thesis of Bell (1976) which he later modified to take account of the growth of the ICTs and related occupations to become the 'information society' thesis (Bell, 1980). Freidson (1973) theory of the professions is based on the post-industrial thesis. Fortunately, for the present analysis, the concept of medical dominance can stand independently of the wider professionalization theme of the post-industrialisation thesis. As Johnson (1973) has pointed out, such status and influence was the outcome of the professional monopolies legally established in the nineteenth century.

The second scenario is derived from the Marx's proletarianization thesis which was updated in the now classic work of Braverman (1974). In this version the assumption is that there is only one management labour strategy and that is to exert direct control over the workforce whether by scientific management, Fordist production techniques or automation. Moreover, the development of information technologies has made possible the means of controlling more directly the work of white-collar, technical and professional work generally. In this way the prognosis is that doctors, nurses and computer specialists too are vulnerable to deskilling and proletarianization. It was Oppenheimer (1973), however, who applied the logic of the argument specifically to professional work and argued that growing bureaucratization is leading to the proletarianization of professional work. This interpretation has, subsequently, been modified by Larson (1980) and Derber (1982) and Derber et al. (1990) in connection with professions within the US (see also Chapter 2). These researchers conclude that despite there being rationalising processes at work the evidence the professions are resistant to the corrosive effects on their autonomy. They manage to do this, firstly, by continuing to control the accreditation of college and university courses. Secondly, by retaining autonomy over the work situation - even if this is now more narrowly defined. Thirdly, members of the professions are often in managerial control of the professional bureaucracies such as hospitals, law firms and accountancy firms. Derber et al (1990) refers to these as logocracies to distinguish them from managerialist firms.

Johnson (1977), in a useful (i.e. classic) article entitled 'Professions in the class structure', contrasted the two 'antithetical theses' (ibid.) of Freidson (1973) and Oppenheimer (1973). His conclusions were based on the Jamous and Peloilles' (1970) 'technicity/indetermination' ratio (see Chapter 2) which enables one to distinguish between different types of knowledge and technical workers. Some professions, particularly with a technical/technological base - such as systems analysts and programmers will be vulnerable to a worsening of their work and market situations (proletarianization) consequent on technological and organizational rationalization. On the other hand, other professional occupations, including doctors, will not be. Their knowledge/power base is far less susceptible to external control and rationalization (although it is certainly not immune). In a recent revamping of this thesis Johnson (1995) has pressed Foucault into service to argue that 'The professions ... are involved in the constitution of the objects of politics; in the identification of new social problems, the construction of the means or instrumentalities for solving them, as well as in staffing the organizations created to cope with them' (ibid., p.23). In this form the autonomous professions are intrinsic to the modern social formations.

In the reconfiguration of health care services the health professions have been engaged in all these activities identified by Johnson. These are, in part, social constructions designed to render 'a realm of affairs *governable*' (ibid., *emphasis in original*). In the case of health care it is the medical profession who has played this role more than any other among the health care professions.

On how to avoid being anachronic

One of the problems of writing any book on IT and healthcare computing is that it can appear 'out of date' even before it is published. The rapid pace of technological change will ensure this is so even if this is as much a consequence of the instability of actor networks and the problems of 'closure'. There are technologies that have not been included until this point which are beginning to be routinely used in hospitals. A good example of this is the growth of document imaging processing (DIP) technologies (e.g. WORM) in the area of electronic patient records (Gay, 1991; Brown and Patrick, 1992; Troll, 1995). These are systems that use scanners to translate writing, print and images into digitilized code that can be entered and stored directly onto a computer system. This ability would appear to offer the possibility of technologically overcoming the problems associated with the automation of medical records. Simply by scanning the paper documents it becomes possible to rapidly 'computerize' the historic records which can then be integrated with other of the hospital data-bases such as the master patient index (Troll, 1995, p.39). Moreover, these systems can play an important part in the multi-media integration of medical imaging (e.g. computerized tomography and radiography, magnetic resonance imaging [MRI], digital angiography, positron emission tomography [PET], and single photon emission CT) with clinical information and data which then forms the basis of the clinical workstation (ibid.). Thus clinicians can access immediately the whole range of patients' information and data. These work station systems are intended by the Information Management Group (IMG) of the NHS Management Executive to interface with the wider hospital systems networks including HISS (Smith and Gunner, 1994). This policy of creating 'fully functioning integrated clinical workstation' has been insightfully described by one doctor as 'the holy grail of every hospital' (Fitzpatrick quoted in Brown and Patrick, 1992, p.10) which might be a cliché but is accurate in its implication, i.e. technologically-led approaches to automating medical records are fraught with problems most of which are not technical. As another interested observer (Project Manager for Hewlett-Packard) has pointed out '[a]n electronic patient record (EPR) must be able to reflect the full complexity of the clinical healthcare process itself, or it will inevitably fail' (Troll, 1995, p.37). As a replacement to the tradition medical records folders they potentially offer a radical extension to the computer-based systems described earlier in Chapter 5 (Smallman, 1992).

This newer digitilized technology may be capable of overcoming the problems of medical-user resistance experienced previously. Indeed, it might be anticipated because of its greater flexibility, particularly in the way information (including visual images) and data is captured. Most of this, however, is surmise and progress to date has been slow and insufficient to provide complete reassurance to hospital managers and professionals that their introduction will provide the solution to the full automation of hospital systems (see Brown and Patrick, 1992). Therefore, while it is possible that these systems will overcome the resistance of doctors to routine use of IT this will be because the technology has been subordinated to the social and organizational imperatives healthcare delivery and not the other way around. This has been a central argument of this book and one which will be revisited in the next section.

The social construction of healthcare computing?

There have been two strands to the argument developed within this book which will be summarised in this section. The first was that IT systems within hospitals are more accurately to be thought of the outcomes of professional-managerial and inter-professional conflicts and not some technological rationality. The second and related strand is that IT systems function well only when they provide the help doctors, nurses and managers believe they need to carry out their work effectively.

In dealing with the issues associated with the first strand it was the social constructionist approach that provided the overall framework for explaining the occupational and managerial dynamics of hospital computer systems. The detailed analysis drew on three main sources: labour process theory, actor network theory and post-bureaucratic organizational theory. Whilst a principal focus of the analysis has been the role IT has played in the changing the patterns of organizational and occupational control (and therefore rooted in a labour process discourse) this was insufficient for a comprehensive analysis that took the technology seriously too. Similarly, actor network theory was insufficient in itself to account for labour processes and professionalism. My eclecticism is derived from a precept set by Abercrombie and Urry who 'worr[ied] less about which discourse [was] privileged ... and more about the manner in which an adequate theory ... [could] be constructed' (1983, p.91). This was something that was relatively easy to achieve in the discussion on post-bureaucratic organizational theory but these models lacked the specificity necessary to deal fully with either the IT systems or the work situations of the professions. Consequently, further detail is required here.

The eclecticism was more apparent than real for the analysis was embedded within an overarching Foucauldian post-structuralism. Moreover, the separate discourses themselves exhibited tendencies that made the potential for integration easier to accomplish. Firstly, in post-Braverman labour process analyses the different 'types of control' (Friedman, 1977; Edwards. 1979) and 'regimes' (Burawoy, 1985) could be viewed as broadly compatible with a Foucauldian model of power (Knights, 1990; Knights and Vurdubakis, 1994). It was noted, however, that the labour process theorists have tended to assume that the 'contested terrain' of work organizations are more economically and materially 'shaped' than does Foucault (1981, p.95): 'Where there is power, there is resistance, and yet, or rather consequently, this resistance is never in a position of exteriority in relation to power'. In the case of the actor network theorists, however, the potential connection stems from the common intellectual debt of Latour, Callon and Foucault to Machiavelli. Whilst, in the discussion of post-bureaucratic organizational forms in Chapter 7 it was the common links with post-structuralist discourse that provided the connections. All of this was more complicated than I had intended but necessary, in my view, to do justice to the complexities of the professional-managerial dynamics that underpin the development of healthcare computing systems within the NHS hospital service.

The second strand, and the one that has taken up most space, has been a sociological review and assessment of healthcare computing and IT within NHS hospitals. The three occupational chapters on computer specialists, doctors and nurses (Chapters 4-6) which examined the interrelation between professionalism, expertise and organizational control were sandwiched between two 'organizational' chapters. The first of these, 'Computers, management strategies and the state' (Chapter 3) was directly concerned with the managerial strategies aspects of healthcare computing and the second 'Hospitals, IT and new organizational forms' (Chapter 7) considered how best to make organizational sense of the new 'internal market' arrangements within the NHS as well as the putative role IT has played in these changes. The shift from technology-led to information-led policies (Chapter 3) and from bureaucratic to post-bureaucratic organizational forms (Chapter 7) provide an underlying rationale to the occupational chapters. The trajectory of technology-led to information-led policies was reflected within the separate chapters on the three key professional groups. Here focus was on the reasons why they each displayed different abilities to influence, or fail to influence, the shape and direction of healthcare computing within hospitals. The chapters also detail, in turn, the various roles IT has played in the reconfiguration of professional autonomy and power within NHS hospitals. In the chapter on nurses (Chapter 6), for instance, IT was explored within the context of the growth of managerialism within nursing and the inter-professional aspects of medical dominance. The most distinctive element within this chapter, however, was the discussion of emotional labour and the implications of the technological rationality of healthcare computing systems. The general conclusion, which applied to doctors too, was that these systems need to accurately reflect the work processes of the potential users as well as the occupational and organizational politics of hospitals if they were to be operationally successful.

At a more general level the overarching claim was that the subordination of computing policies information management has led to an erosion of the boundary between professional autonomy and managerial control within hospitals. Doctors and nurses have become an integral part of the hospital management and not simply members of a skilled and, in the case of doctors, powerful workforce. These changes are a reflection of changes on a broader social canvas in which the established professions are undergoing changes that make it increasingly difficult for them to sustain their 'traditional' independence and pressurising them into an 'organic' integration within the 'service class' (Abercrombie and Urry, 1983, p.147). A shift of emphasis that I have argued corresponds to a particular kind of responsible autonomy (Dent, 1993). In labour process terminology these changes indicated a marked move towards responsible autonomy and away from professional autonomy that reflected an incorporation of these professions (especially doctors) than has ever been previously the case. The computer specialists within the NHS, by contrast, found that their work was no longer defined as core to the enterprise of health care delivery and forced to leave. There did appear to be the possibility that a policy of 'hybridization' might have enabled many to switch to information systems work but in the event this did not happen. Information management became instead a new management specialty based on a different, if related, knowledge and skills base.

Health information systems and the emergence of a professional-managerial cadre

The introduction of information management within the NHS was an integral part of the general strategic changes that swept through the service from the mid 1980s onwards which appeared to suggest that hospitals would become IT-dependent as well as clinically directed organizations. The evidence of the earlier chapters makes it clear that IT has more often been part of a management rhetoric than a technical tool of change. The management information systems that following the Griffith's Inquiry (1983), for instance, were allegedly dependent on IT support yet such support was generally not available (Dent et al, 1991). Similarly, and more recently, IT support has not been available in an adequate and reliable enough form to provide comprehensive support for the new resource management systems even where a HISS strategy has been pursued. Nevertheless, some hospitals do appear to be near attaining the 'holy grail' of an integrated IT system. Possibly the best example is the system at Burton on Trent (Gowing, 1994: Paul, 1995) which apparently includes automated medical records. The general organizational changes, however, did not require that the new IT systems support be complete so long as the rhetoric was sufficiently persuasive to bring about the changes in the roles of doctors and nurses to include responsibilities for budgets. The introduction of resource management and the 'internal market' was not only an attempt to reduce the relative cost of delivering health care but, in the process, one that incorporated doctors directly into the management of hospitals. This contrasted with the pre-existing situation where the relationship could best be described as an accommodation. Now doctors are taking the view that if there has to be financial accountability at hospital level they had best have a central role. Only in this way can they continue to maintain their professional dominance within the more managerialist NHS. In this way they are adapting to the changed organizational arrangements without giving up their autonomy and control over the medical work processes and division of labour.

The nurses' managerial role has also changed and senior nurses too have to pay close attention to costs and efficiencies. They now provide support to the clinical director and responsibility for the resource management and skill mix on the wards. Nurse managers now not only manage their professional colleagues but also a growing number of health care assistants. In addition, the nurse role is being further extended in part as a renewed professionalization project and partly (in the wake of the reduction in junior doctors hours) a response to need to cover tasks previously carried out by junior doctors (Walby et al., 1994, p.12). In terms of the proletarianization and professionalization scenarios, the prognosis for nursing is complex. Clearly the employment of health care assistants represents the deskilling and proletarianization of elements of nursing work (but not necessary nurses). The extension of the clinical nursing role, however, is an ambiguous development and for all its veneer of professionalism it represents, on closer examination, an intensification of work. Moreover, the extended role comprises of tasks that are subject to tightly defined protocols which offer minimal opportunities for professional judgement to be exercised. What is more likely to protect the professional status of nursing is their continued if often ambivalent role relations with doctors in the hospital division of labour.

One specific area of inter-professional activity that may bring nurses and doctors to work more closely together is that of clinical audit. Until recently audit work for the two groups was entirely separate but from 1995 the processes will be integrated and become known as clinical audit. At the same time, the criteria used will be substantially defined by the health authority purchasers (Department of Health, 1994; NHS Management Executive, 1994). This is not to assume that the criteria will necessarily relate to narrowly managerial considerations for they will be based on public health specialists' defined criteria. On the other hand, clinical audit may represent the belief that effective and systematic audits are more likely to occur if nurses become responsible for them than if they remain wholly under the control of doctors. A speculative point, but insofar that it may be true could underpin the nurses' professionalism.

On the managerial side of the equation, as it were, there has emerged a new 'breed' of hospital manager who have a keenness to inculcate new integrative organizational culture into the hospitals. Ones that might incorporate the professional cultures of doctors and nurses. For a few this means directly confronting the tradition of medical dominance. Mike Filby (1995, p.691) illustrated the point well in his review of *Controlling the Health Professions* (Harrison and Pollitt, 1994):

> A recent opinion piece in the *Health Services Journal* enjoined managers to take off the gloves to the 'medical Mafia' in the NHS over job reviews, clinical audit, training in evidence based medicine and indeed PRP in the quest for more efficient use of resources.

But, as Filby goes on to comment, if things were that easy it would already have been done with the introduction of the Griffiths' reforms nearly 10 years ago. Instead, what has happened has been that hospital managers have continued to work closely with doctors in order to ensure they too share in the 'cloak of clinical legitimacy'. This is the way in which professional expertise is currently being rendered governable (Johnson, 1995) which in the NHS has become characterized by more local and particularistic hospital cultures than was previously the case. These are organizational cultures that cut across national and regional professional and management organizations. Doctors now fight for the interests of 'their' hospitals as well as their professional specialty. Nurses are concerned about the future of 'their' hospital and any threat of job losses. This new localised and pragmatic realism is yet another reason why - despite some surface similarities - hospitals are not analogous to franchised 'burger bars' (Ritzer, 1993). These new and complex hospitals are held together, however, less by sophisticated integrated IT systems and more by the organizations' specific systems of values and interests and sustaining these is the key role of the new cadre of hospital management.

Bibliography

Abbott, B. (1985) 'A regional computer strategy'. *British Journal of Health Care Computing (BJHC)*, Vol.2, No.2, May, pp.16-17.

Abercrombie, N. and Urry, J. (1983) *Capital, Labour and the Middle Classes,* Hemel Hempstead: Allen & Unwin.

Adams, I.D., Chan, M., and Clifford, P.C. (1986) 'Computer-aided diagnosis of abdominal pain: a multi-centre study'. *British Medical Journal,* Vol.293, pp.800-4.

Albrow, M. (1970) *Bureaucracy*, London: Macmillan

Amsterdamska, O. (1990) 'Surely you must be joking Monsieur Latour!', *Science Technology and Human Values*, Vol.15, No.4, pp.495-504.

Anderson, J. (1984) 'Clinical records systems - an overview', in B. Kostrewski (ed.) *Current Perspectives in Health Computing*, Cambridge: Cambridge University Press/British Computer Society, pp.107-14.

Anderson, J.G. and Jay, S.J. (1983) 'Utilisation of computers in clinical practice - role of physician networks: preliminary communication', *Journal of the Royal Society of Medicine*, Vol.76, pp.45-52.

Armstrong, P.(1984) 'Competition between the organizational professions and the evolution of management control strategies', in K. Thompson (ed.) *Work, Employment and Unemployment*, Milton Keynes: Open University Press, pp.97-120.

Arluke, A. (1977) 'Social control rituals in medicine', in R. Dingwall, C. Heath, M. Read and M. Stacey (eds), *Health Care and Health Knowledge*, London: Croom Helm, pp.108-25.

Atkinson, C. and Peel ,V. (1992) 'New Breed' *BJHC*, Vol.9, No.1, pp.17 and 28.

Audit Commission (1991) *The virtue of patients - making use of ward nursing resources.* London HMSO.

________. (1992a) *Caring systems: a handbook for managers of nursing and project managers,* London: HMSO.

________. (1992b) *Making time for patients,* London: HMSO.

________. (1995a) *For Your Information: a study of information management and system in the acute hospital*, London: HMSO.
________. (1995b) *Setting the Records Straight*, London: HMSO.
Barber, B. and Abbott, W. (1972) *Computing and Operational Research at the London Hospital*. London: Butterworths.
Barker, J. and Downing, H. (1985) 'Word processing and the transformation of patriarchal relations in the control in the office', in D. MacKenzie and J. Wacjman (eds) *The Social Shaping of Technology*, Buckingham: Open University Press, pp.147-64.
Barnett, G.O. (1968,) 'Computers in patient care', *New England Journal of Medicine*, Vol.279, No.24, pp.1321-7.
________. (1982) 'The computer and clinical judgment', *New England Journal of Medicine*, Vol.307, No.8, pp.493-4.
Barnet, G.O., Winickoff, R., Dorsey, J.L., Morgan, M.M., and Lurie, R.S. (1978) 'Quality assurance through automated monitoring and concurrent feedback using a computer-based medical information system', *Medical Care*, Vol.XVI, No.11, pp.962-70.
Barnett, G.O., Justice, N.S., Somand, M.E., Adams, J.B., Waxman, B.D., Beaman, P.D., Parent, M.S., Van Deusan, F.R. and Greenlie, J.K. (1979) 'A computer-based medical information system for ambulatory care', *Proceedings of the IEEE*, Vol.67, No.9, pp.1226-37.
Baudrillard, J. (1975) *The Mirror of Production.*, St Louis: Telos Press.
________. (1983) *Simulations*, New York, Semitext(e).
Bauman, Z. (1992) *Intimations of Postmodernity* London: Routledge.
Berger, P.L. and Luckman, T. (1971) *The Social Construction of Reality*, Harmondsworth: Penguin.
Bell, D. (1973) *The Coming of Post-Industrial Society: a venture in social forecasting*, New York: Basic Books.
________. (1980) 'The social framework of the Information Society', in T. Forester (ed.) *The Microelectronics Revolution*, Oxford: Blackwell.
Bijker, W.E., Hughes, T.P. and Pinch, T.J. (eds) (1987) *The Social Construction of Technological Systems*, MIT Press: London.
Bittner, E. and Garfinkel, H. (1967) '"Good" organizational reasons for "bad" clinic records', in H. Garfinkel (ed.) *Studies in Ethnomethodology* , New Jersey: Prentice Hall, pp.186-207.
Björkman, J.W. (1989) 'Politicizing medicine and medicalizing politics: physician power in the United States', in G. Freddi and J.W. Björkman (eds) *Controlling Medical Professional: the comparative politics of health governance*, Sage: London, pp.28-73.
Bjorn-Anderson, N. and Rasmussen, L.F.B.(1980) 'Sociological Implications of Computer Systems', in H. T. Smith and T. R. G. Green (eds) *Human Interaction with Computers*, London: Academic Press, pp.97-123.
Bloomfield, B.P.(1995) 'Power, Machines and Social Relations: delegating to information technology in the National Health Service', *Organization*, Vol.2, No.3/4, pp.489-518.

Bloomfield, B.P. and Coombs, R. (1992) 'Information technology, control and power: the centralization and decentralization debate revisited' *Journal of Management Studies* , Vol.29, No.4, pp.459-84.
Bloomfield, B.P., Coombs, R.W., Cooper, D.J. and Rea, D.M. (1990) 'The Resource Management Initiative in the NHS: the translation of an "accounting" system'. *Final Report to the Leverhulme Trust*, CROMTEC, UMIST. August.
Bloomfield, B.P., Coombs, R., Cooper, D.J. and Rea, D. (1992) 'Machines and manoeuvres: responsibility accounting and the construction of hospital information systems', *Accounting Management and Information Technology*, Vol.2, No.4, pp.197-219.
Bloor, M. (1976a) 'Professional autonomy and client exclusion: a study in ENT clinics', in M. Wadsworth and D. Robinson (eds) *Studies in Everyday Medical Life*. London: Martin Robertson, pp.52-67.
________. (1976b) 'Bishop Berkeley and the adenotonsillectomy enigma: an exploration in the social construction of medical disposals'. *Sociology*, Vol.10, No.1, pp.43-62.
Boas, M. and Chain, S. (1976) *Big Mac: the unauthorized story of McDonald's*, New York: Dutton.
Boguslaw, R. (1965) *The New Utopians: a study of system design and social change*, Englewood Cliffs, NJ: Prentice-Hall
Boje, D. M. and Dennehy, R. F. (1993) *Managing in the Postmodern World*, Dubuque, Iowa: Kendall/Hunt Publishing Co.
Björkman, J. W. (1989) 'Politicizing medicine and medicalizing politics: physician power in the US', in G. Freddi and J.W. Björkman eds) *Controlling Medical Professionals: the comparative politics of health governance*. London: Sage, pp.28-73.
Bosk, C.L. (1979) *Forgive and Remember: managing medical failure*, London: University of Chicago Press.
Bradburn, C., Zeleznikow, J. Adams, A. (1993) 'FLORENCE: synthesis of case-based and model-based reasoning in a nursing care planning system.' *Computers in Nursing*, Vol.11, No.1, pp.20-4.
Braverman, H. (1974) *Labor and Monopoly Capital*, London: Monthly Review Press.
British Computer Society (1990) 'From potential to reality: 'hybrids' a critical force in the application of IT in the 1990s', *Report by the British Computer Society Task Group on Hybrids*, London: The British Computer Society.
The British Journal of Healthcare Computing (*BJHC*) (1984) 'Körner implementation gets backing from government', Vol.1, No.2, p.5.
________. (1985a) 'Fairey's way forward', Vol.2, No.2, pp.7-9.
________. (1985b) 'Information Advisory Group developments', Vol.2, No.4, p.8.
________. (1985c) 'Developments: Inter-Regional Consortium/ International Computers Ltd to upgrade PAS', Vol.2, No.4, p.7.
________. (1986) 'Fairey's framework' Vol.3, No.3. pp.12-13.

________. (1987) 'Regional networks', Vol.4, No.6, p.7.
________. (1988a) 'IRC under pressure', Vol.5, No.10, p.3.
________. (1988b) 'CFM establishes Wessex company', Vol.5, No.7, p.3.
________. (1989a) 'Regions take steps to devolve computer units' Vol.6, No.3, p.5.
________. (1989b) 'Noose tightens for RHA computing' Vol.6, No.4, p.4.
________. (1989c) 'NHS to sell UK's biggest health IT team', Vol.6, No.1, p.6.
________. (1989d) 'West Midlands buy-out goes ahead' Vol.6, No.7, p.7.
________. (1989e) 'West Midlands in talks with HBO' Vol.6, No.6, p.3.
________. (1989f) 'West Midlands buy-out goes ahead' Vol.6, No.10, p.7.
________. (1989g) 'IRC fulfils its new purpose' Vol.6, No.3, p.5.
________. (1989h) 'West Midlands seeks new partners' Vol.6, No.8, p.3.
________. (1989l) £0.5bn for HISS implementation', Vol6, No.4, p.3.
________. (1990a) 'New RMI sites announced', Vol.7, No.1, p.4.
________. (1990b) 'QA falls at first' Vol.7, No.2, p.9.
________. (1990c) 'Shopping for FM' Vol.7, No.1, p.17.
________. (1990d) 'Redundant QA staff find a home from home with Hoskyns' Vol.7, No.6, p.6.
________. (1990e) 'Oracle and Qa in joint venture' Vol.7, No.5, p.5.
________. (1990f) 'Government auditors condemn NHS IT management and call for "sustained action"' Vol.7, No.10, pp.8-9.
________. (1991a) 'Row looming over future development of IRC PAS' Vol.8, No.2, p.9.
________. (1991b) 'Future of IRC PAS still uncertain' Vol.8, No.3, p.6.
________. (1991c) 'IRC PAS development goes to ICL' Vol.8, No.8, p.2.
________. (1991d) 'NHS loses following Qa collapse' Vol.8, No.9, p.2.
________. (1993) 'NHS gets professional IT group' Vol.10, No.4, pp.4-5.
The British Journal of Healthcare Computing & Information Management (BJHC & IM) (1994a) 'ICL gets 25 year IRC PAS licence', Vol.11, No.1, pp.4-5.
________. (1994b) 'Report says unhappy PAS users will spend £100m on new systems', Vol.11, No.1, p.6.
________. (1995a) 'Audit Commission says IT problems perpetuated by poor management', Vol.12, No.7, pp.4-5.
________. (1995b) 'Concerning reports', Vol.12, No.7, p.9.
British Medical Journal *Supplement* (1977), 'Submission of Evidence' 29th January, p.301 (para.2.5) and p.303 (para.3.12).
Brittain, J.M. (1992) 'The emerging market for information professionals in the UK National Health Service', *International Journal of Information Management*, Vol.12, pp.261-71.
Brown, P.(1993) 'Regional computer centres: shaping up or shipping out?' *The BJHC & IM*, Vol.10, No.8, pp.21-2.
Brown, R.K. (1992) *Understanding Industrial Organisations*, London, Routledge.

Brown, P. and Patrick, M. (1992) 'Imaging the complete medical record', *BJHC*, Vol.9, No.8, pp.9-10.
Buchanan, A. (1993) 'Computerised care plans in Tayside' *Nursing Standard*, Vol.7, No.26 (17 Mar), pp.37-9).
Buchanan, D.A. (1983) 'Technological imperatives and strategic choice', in G. Winch (ed.) *Information Technology in Manufacturing Processes*, London: Rossendale, pp.72-80.
________. (1986) 'Management objectives in technical change', in D. Knights and H. Willmott (eds) *Managing the Labour Process*, Aldershot: Gower, pp.67-84.
Buchanan, D.A. and Boddy, D. (1983) *Organizations in the Computer Age: technological imperatives and strategic choice*, Aldershot: Gower.
Bullas, S. (1989) *Case Mix Management System: core specification* Resource Management, Department of Health: London.
Burawoy, M. (1979) *Manufacturing Consent: changes in the labour process under capitalism*, Chicago: University of Chicago Press.
________. (1985) *The Politics of Production: factory regimes under capitalism and socialism*, London: Verso.
Burgess, R.G. (1984) *In the Field: an introduction to field research*, London: Allen & Unwin.
Burnett, G.J. and Nolan, R.L. (1975) 'At last, major roles for mini computers', *Harvard Business Review*, Vol.53, No.2, pp.148-56.
Burns, T. (1969) 'On the plurality of social systems' in T. Burns (ed.) *Industrial Man*, Harmondsworth: Penguin, pp.232-49.
Burns, T. and Stalker, G.M. (1961) *The Management of Innovation,* London: Tavistock.
Burrell, G. and Morgan, G. (1979) *Sociological Paradigms and Organisational Analysis,* London: Heinemann. ok
Burrows, R. and Loader, B. (eds) (1994) *Towards a Post-Fordist Welfare State?* London Routledge.
Butler, J. R. and Vaile, M. S. B. (1984) *Health and Health Services,* London: Routledge and Kegan Paul.
Bylinsky, G. (1980) 'Here comes the second computer revolution', in T. Forester (ed.) *The Microelectronics Revolution*, Oxford: Blackwell, pp.3-15.
Bywater, M. and Wilkins, C. (1995) 'Good reading for a small price: view from the bridge' *BJHC & IM*, Vol.12, No.7, p.10.
Caddick, P.T. and Lee, D.T. (1974) 'The planning and control of health care computing policy', in J. Anderson and J. M. Forsythe (eds) , *Stockholm, August 5-10*, Oxford: North-Holland, pp.39-44.
Callon, M. (1986) 'Some elements of a sociology of translation: domestication of the scallops and the fishermen of St Brieuc Bay', in J. Law (ed.) *Power, Action and Belief: a new sociology of knowledge?* London: Routledge and Kegan Paul, pp.196-233.
Callon, M. (1987) 'Society in the making: the study of technology as a tool for sociological analysis', in W.E. Bijker, T.P. Hughes and T.J. Pinch, T.

J. (eds) *The Social Construction of Technological Systems* MIT Press: London, pp.83-103.
Callon, M. and Latour, B. (1981) 'Unscrewing the big Leviathan: how actors macro-structure reality and how sociologists help them to do so', in K. Knorr-Cetina and A.V. Cicourel (eds) *Advances in Social Theory and Methodology: towards an integration of micro- and macro-sociologies.* London: Routledge and Kegan Paul, pp.277-303.
Callon, M. and Law, J. (1982) 'On interests and their transformation', *Social Studies of Science*, Vol.1, pp.615-25.
Campbell, J.R., Seelig, C.B., Wigton, R.S. Givner, N., Patil, K. and Tape, T.G. (1988) 'Clinic function and computerized ambulatory records: a concurrent study with conventional records', R.A. Green (ed.) *Proceedings: Annual Symposium on Computer Applications in Medical Care,* Long Beach, California: IEEE Computer Society Press.
Cane, A. (1988) 'Advisers at board level', *Financial Times*, 5 October.
Checkland, P.B. (1981) *Systems Thinking, Systems Practice* Chichester: John Wiley.
Checkland, P.B. and Scholes, J. (1991) *Soft Systems Methodology in Action* , Chichester: John Wiley.
Child, J. (1985) 'Management strategies, new technology and the labour process', in D. Knights, H. Willmott and D. Collinson.(eds) *Job Redesign: Critical Perspectives on the Labour Process,* Aldershot: Gower, pp.107-41.
________. (1986) 'New technology and the service class', in K. Purcell, S. Wood, A. Waton and S. Allen (eds) *The Changing Experience of Employment: restructuring and recession*, Basingstoke: Macmillan.
Clark, P. and Staunton, N. (1989) *Innovation in Technology and Organization*, London: Routledge.
Clarkson, D. (1991) 'Artificial solutions?' *British Journal of Healthcare Computing* Vol.8, No.9 (November). pp.15-16
Clegg, S.R. (1989) *Frameworks of Power*, London: Sage.
________. (1990) *Modern Organizations: organization studies in the postmodern world.* London: Sage.
Clegg, S. and Dunkerley (1980) *Organization, Class and Control* London: Routledge and Kegan Paul.
Cochrane, A.(1971) *Effectiveness and Efficiency*, London: NPHT.
Cockburn, C. (1985) 'The material of male power', in D. Mackenzie and J. Wajcman (eds) *The Social Shaping of Technology* . Milton Keynes: Open University Press, pp.125-46.
Coleman, J. S., Katz, E. and Menzel, H. (1966) *Medical Innovation: a diffusion study*, Indianapolis: Bobbs-Merrill.
Collingridge, D. (1990) 'Technology organisation and incrementalism: the space shuttle' *Technology Analysis and Strategic Management* Vol.2, No.2, pp.181-200.
Computer Weekly (1990a) 'Hospital project hit by withdrawal of bidders', 22 February, p.19.

________. (1990b) 'Poor IT management threatens NHS reforms', 29 November, p.13.
Coombs, R. and Cooper, D. (1992) 'Accounting for Patients? in R. Loveridge and K. Starkey (eds)*Continuity and Crisis in the NHS* , Buckingham: Open University Press, pp.118-25.
Coombs, R. and Jonsson, O. (1991) 'New technology and management in a non-market environment: a case study of office automation in Swedish hospitals', in C. Smith, D. Knights and H. Willmott (eds) *White-Collar Work: the non-manual labour process*, Basingstoke: Macmillan, pp.89-107.
Cooper, R. (1989) 'Modernism, postmodernism and organizational analysis 3: the contribution of Jacques Derrida" *Organizational Studies* Vol 10, No.4: 479-82.
Cooper, R. and Burrell, G. (1988) 'Modernism, postmodernism and organizational analysis: an introduction' *Organizational Studies* Vol.9, No.1: 91-112.
Cousins, C. (1986) 'The labour process in the state welfare sector', in D. Knights and H. Willmott (eds) *Managing the Labour Process*, Aldershot: Gower, pp.85-108.
Covaski, M.A. and Dirsmith, M.W. (1983) 'Budgeting as a means for control and loose-coupling' *Accounting, Organizations and Society,* Vol.8, No.4, pp.323-40.
Cox, D. (1991) 'Health service management - a sociological view: Griffiths and the non-negotiated order of the hospital', in J. Gabe, M. Calnan and M. Bury (eds) *The Sociology of the Health Service*. London: Routledge, pp.89-114.
________. (1992) 'Crisis and opportunity in health service management', in R. Loveridge and K. Starkey (eds) *Continuity and Crisis in the NHS*, Buckingham: Open University Press, pp.23-42.
Cross, M. (1993a) 'Information for purchasers: a WAN-dering we will go', *Health Service Journal*, 27 May, pp.35-8.
________. (1993b) 'Hospital Information Systems: HISSSSSSS-BANG!' *Health Service Journal*, 17 June, pp.39-47.
________. (1994) 'The generation gap'. *Health Services Journal, IT update,* 26th May, pp.4-6.
________. (1995) 'No longer counting beans', *Health Services Journal, IT Update,* 26th January: p.1.
Crow, G. (1989) 'The use of the concept of 'strategy' in recent sociological literature' *Sociology*, Vol.23, No.1, pp.1-24.
Davies, C. (1992) 'Gender, history and management style in nursing: towards a theoretical synthesis', in M. Savage and A. Witz (eds) *Gender and Bureaucracy*, Oxford: Blackwell, pp.229-52.
Davies, C. and Rosser, J. (1986) 'Gendered Jobs in the Health Service: a problem for labour process analysis', in D. Knights and H. Willmott (eds) *Gender and the Labour Process*, .Aldershot: Gower, pp.94-116.

Davis, R. Buchanan, B. and Shortliffe, E. (1977) 'Production rules as a representation for a knowledge-based consultation program', *Artificial Intelligence*, Vol.8, pp.15-45.

de Dombal, F.T., Leaper, D.J., Staniland, J.R. (1972) 'Computer-aided diagnosis of acute abdominal pain', *British Medical Journal*, Vol.2, pp.9-13.

de Dombal, F.T. and Horrocks, J.C. (1974) 'Computer-aided diagnosis: conclusions from an overall experience involving 4469 patients', in J. Anderson and J.M. Forsythe (eds) *MEDINFO 1974: Proceedings of the First World Conference on Medical Informatics, Stockholm, August 5-10*, Oxford: North-Holland, pp.581-5

de Dombal, F.T. (1991) 'The diagnosis of acute abdominal pain with computer assistance: worldwide perspective' *Annales de Chirurgie* Vol.45, No 4: 273-7.

Dent, M. (1985) *Doctors and the development of hospital computer systems.* (End of Award Report No.GOO 230077) (1st May). London: Economic and Social Research Council.

________. (1989) *Doctors and Computers*, Unpublished Ph.D. thesis, Coventry: University of Warwick.

________. (1990a) 'Organizations and change in renal work: a study of the impact of a computer system within two hospitals' *Sociology of Health and Illness,* Vol 12, No.4 (Dec.), pp.413-31

________. (1991) 'Information technology and managerial strategies in the NHS: computer strategies, organizational change and the labour process' *Critical Perspectives on Accounting,* Vol.2, pp.331-60.

________. (1993) 'Professionalism, educated labour and the state: hospital medicine and the new managerialism' *The Sociological Review* Vol.41, No.2, pp.244-73

________. (1995a) 'Doctors, peer review and quality assurance.' In T. Johnson, G. Larkin and M. Saks (eds) *Health Professions in Europe.* London: Routledge. pp.86-102.

________. (1995b) 'The new National Health Service: a case of postmodernism?' *Organization Studies,* Vol.16, No.5, pp.875-99.

Dent, M., Green, R., Smith, J.J., and Cox, D. (1992) 'Modes of innovation in management information systems', in R. Loveridge and K. Starkey (eds) *Continuity and Crisis in the National Health Service*, Milton Keynes: Open University Press, pp.126-45.

Denzin, N.K. (1978) *The Research Act: a theoretical introduction to sociological methods.* (second edition), New York: McGraw-Hill.

Department of Health and Social Security (DHSS) (1972) *Management Arrangements for the Reorganised National Health Service*, London: HMSO.

________. (1977) *Interim Report on the Evaluation of the National Health Service Experimental Computer Programme*, London.

________. (1982) *The Evaluation of the NHS Computer R & D Programme: An Analysis of Performance Criteria Measurement Results.*

Review Paper on Computer Evaluation for the Evaluation Working Group, (June), London.
________. (1986) Circular HN (86) 34, *Health Services Management: Resource Management (Management Budgeting) in Health Authorities*, London.
Department of Health (1990) *Training for Information Management Staff*, London: Department of Health.
________. (1993) *Clinical Audit: meeting and improving standards in health care*. London: Department of Health.
________. (1994) *The Evolution of Clinical Audit* Heywood, Lancs: The Health Publications Unit.
Derber, C. (1982) 'The proletarianization of the professional: a review essay', in C. Derber (ed.) *Professions as Workers: mental labor in advanced capitalism*, Boston, Mass.: Hall and Co, pp.13-34.
Derber, C., Schwartz, W.A. and Magrass, Y. (1990) *Power in the Highest Degree: professionals and the rise of a new mandarin order*, New York and Oxford: Oxford University Press.
Derrida, J. (1978) *Writing and Difference*, London: Routledge and Kegan Paul.
Derrida, J. (1981) *Positions*, Chicago, Ill: University Press.
Dick, R.S. and Steen, E.B. (eds) (1991)*The Computer-Based Patient Record*. Washington, D.C.: National Academy Press.
Dickson, G. W. and Wetherbe, J.C. (1985) *The Management of Information Systems*, London: McGraw Hill.
Döhler, M. (1989) 'Physicians' professional autonomy in the welfare state: endangered or preserved?' in *Controlling Medical Professionals: the comparative politics of health governance*. G. Freddi and J.W. Björkman (eds), London: Sage. pp.178-97.
Donabedian, A. (1966) 'Evaluating the Quality of Medical Care' *Milbank Fund Quarterly*, Vol.64, No 3, Part 2, pp.166-206.
Dreyfus, H. and Dreyfus, S. (1989) 'Why computers may never think like people', in Forester, T. (ed.) *Computers in the Human Context: Information Technology and People*. Oxford: Blackwell, pp.125-43.
Eames, S. (1989) 'Hospital Information Support Systems: the Greenwich experience' *BJHC*, Vol.6, No.9, pp.9-11.
Earl, M.J. (1989)*Management Strategies for Information Technology*, Hemel Hempstead: Prentice Hall.
Earl, M.J. and Skyrme, D.J. (1992) Hybrid managers - what do we know about them?', *Journal of Information Systems*, Vol.2, pp.169-87.
Edwards, J.S. (1991) *Building Knowledge-Based Systems: towards a methodology*, London: Pitman.
Edwards, R. (1979) *Contested Terrain: the transformation of the workplace in the twentieth century*, London: Heinemann.

Eldridge, J.E.T. (1973) *The Sociology of Industrial Life* London: Nelson
Elger, A. J. (1975) 'Industrial organizations - a processual perspective', in J. B. McKinley (ed.) *Processing People: cases in organizational behaviour*, London: Holt, Rinehart and Winston, pp.91-149.
Elias, N. (1978) *What is Sociology?* London: Hutchinson.
Ellison, D. L. (1978) *The Bio Medical Fix*, Connecticut: Greenwood.
Elster, J. (1982) 'Marxism, functionalism and game theory, the case of methodological individualism', *Theory and Society*, Vol.11, pp.453-82.
________. (1989) *Nuts and Bolts for Social Sciences*, Cambridge: Cambridge University Press.
Elston, M. A (1991) 'The politics of professional power: medicine in a changing health service', in J. Gabe, M. Calnan and M. Bury (eds) *The Sociology of the Health Service,* London: Routledge, pp.58-88.
Enthoven, A.C. (1985) *Reflections on the Management of the NHS,* NPHT, London.
Erickson, K.T. and Gilbertson, D.E. (1969) 'Case records in the mental hospital', in S. Wheeler (ed.) *On Record: files and dossiers in American life*, New York: Sage, pp.389-412.
Fagin, C.M. (1992) 'Cost-effectiveness of Nursing Care Revisited: 1981-90', in L. Aitken and C. Fagin (eds) *Charting Nursing's Future: agenda for the 1990s* . London: J.B. Lippincott & Co. pp.13-28.
Featherstone, M. (1991) *Consumer Culture and Postmodernism*. London: Sage.
Feigenbaum, E.A. and McCorduck, P.(1984) *The Fifth Generation: artificial intelligence and Japan's computer challenge of the world*, London: Pan Books.
Fiddleman, R.H. (1980) 'Proliferation of COSTAR: a status report' , in J.T. O'Neill (ed.) *Proceedings of the Fourth Annual Symposium on Computer Applications in Medical Care*. Long Beach, California:IEEE, PP.1-4.
Fieschi, M. (1990) *Artificial Intelligence in Medicine: Expert Systems*. London: Chapman and Hall.
Filby, M. (1995) [Book review] 'S. Harrison and C. Pollitt, *Controlling Health Professionals: The Future of Work and Organizations in the NHS,* Buckingham: Open University Press, 1994', *Sociology of Health and Illness,* Vol.5, No.17, pp.691-2. .
Fineman, S. (1994) 'Organizing and emotion: towards a social construction.' In J. Hassard and M. Parker (eds) *Towards a New Theory of Organizations*. London: Routledge. pp.75-86.
Fischer, P.J.; Stratman, W.C.; Lundsgarde, H.P.; and Steele, D.J. (1980) 'User reaction to PROMIS: issues related to acceptability of medical innovation', in J.T. O'Neill (ed.) *Proceedings of the Fourth Annual Symposium on Computer Applications in Medical Care*, Long Beach, California: IEEE, pp.1722-30.
Fitter, M. and Sime, M. (1980) 'Creating responsive computers: responsibility and shared decision-making', in H.T. Smith and T.R.G.

Green (eds) *Human Interaction with Computers* London: Academic Press, pp.39-66.
Fitter, M.J. and Cruikshank, J. (1983) 'Doctors using computers: a case study', in M.E. Sime and M.J. Coombs (eds) *Designing for Human-Computer Communication*, London: Academic Press, pp.239-60.
Flynn, R. (1992) *Structures of Control in Health Management*, London: Routledge.
Foot, M. (1973) *Aneurin Bevan* (Vol.2), David-Poynter: London.
Forester, T. (1987) *High-Tech Society*, Oxford: Blackwell.
Foucault, M. (1977) *Discipline and Punish.: the birth of the prison,* Harmondsworth: Allen Lane/Penguin.
________. (1981) *The History of Sexuality. Volume one: an introduction,* Harmondsworth: Penguin. ok
Fox, A. (1974) *Beyond Contract: work power and trust relations,* London: Faber and Faber.
Fox, J. (1977) 'Medical computing and the user', *International Journal of Man-Machine Studies*, Vol.9, p.669-686.
________. (1979) 'Developments of hospital computing', *Journal of the Royal Society of Medicine*, Vol.72, pp.425-31.
Freddi, G. and Björkman, J.W. (1989) *Controlling Medical Professionals: the comparative politics of health governance.* London: Sage.
Freidson, E. (1970) *Medical Dominance.* New York: Atherton Press.
________. (1973) 'Professionalisation and the organisation of middle-class labour in post-industrial society', *Sociological Review Monograph*, No. 20.
________. (1975) *Doctoring Together: a study of professional social control*, Oxford: Elsevier.
________. (1976) 'The development of administration accountability in health services', *American Behavioural Scientist*, Vol.19, No.3, pp.286-98.
Friedman, A.L. (1977) *Industry and Labour* London: Macmillan.
Friedman, A.L. and Greenbaum, J. (1984) 'Wanted: renaissance people', *Datamation,* 1 September, pp.134-44.
Friedman, A.L. with Cornford, D.S. (1989) *Computer Systems Development: history, organization and implementation* Chichester: Wiley.
Friedman, R.B. and Gustafson, D.H. (1977) 'Computers in clinical medicine, a critical review', in *Computers and Biomedical Research*, Vol.10, pp.199-204.
Gallagher, E. B. (1977) 'Home dialysis and socio-medical policy', in M. Stacey, M. Reid, C. Heath and R. Dingwall (eds) *Health and the Division of Labour*, London: Croom Helm. pp.63-85.
Galliers, R. D. and Sutherland, A.R. (1991) 'Information systems management and strategy formulation: the "stages of growth" model revisited', *Journal of Information Systems,* Vol.1, pp.89-114.

Garfinkel, H. (ed) (1967) *Studies in Ethnomethodology,* . New Jersey: Prentice Hall.

Gay, K. (1991) 'Altered Images', *BJHC,* VOL.8, No.6, pp.14-15.

Gedrych, D.A. (1970) 'The Department's policy and objectives', in M. E. Abrams (ed.) *Medical Computing: progress and problems*, London: Chatto and Windus/British Computer Society.

Gerhardt, U. (1987) 'Parsons, role theory, and health interaction.' In G. Scambler (ed.) *Sociological Theory and Medical Sociology*. London: Tavistock. pp.111-33.

Gibson, C. F. and R. L. Nolan (1974) 'Managing the four stages of EDP growth', *Harvard Business Review,* January-February, pp.76-88.

Giddens, A. (1984) *The Constitution of Society: outline of the theory of structuration,* Cambridge: Polity Press.

________. (1987) *Social Theory and Modern Sociology*, Cambridge, Polity Press.

________. (1990) *The Consequences of Modernity*, Cambridge: Polity.

________. (1994) *Beyond Left and Right: the future of radical politics*, Cambridge: Polity.

Giebink, G. A. and Hurst, L. L. (1975) *Computers Projects in Health Care*, University of Michigan, Anne Arbor: Health Administration Press.

Godber, G. (1976) 'The confidential enquiry into maternal deaths. A limited study of clinical results', in G. McLachlan (ed.) *A Question of Quality? roads to assurance in medical care,* London: NPHT/Oxford University Press, pp.23-34.

Goffman, E. (1972) *Interaction Ritual*, London: Allen Lane.

Goldsmith, O. and Mason, A. (eds) (1974) *Information for Action*, Joint Working Party on the Organisation of Medical Work in Hospitals, London: DHSS.

Goldthorpe, J.H. (1982) 'On the service class, its formation and future', in A. Giddens and G. Mackenzie (eds) *Social Class and the Division of Labour*, Cambridge: Cambridge University Press.

Gough, I. (1979) *The Political Economy of the Welfare State*, London: Macmillan.

Gowing, W. (1994) 'Operational systems' in J. Keen (ed.) *Information Management in Health Services*, Buckingham: Open University Press, pp.31-49.

Greenbaum, J. (1976) 'Division of labour in the computer field', *Monthly Review*, Vol.28, No.3, pp.40-55.

Greener, B. (1989) 'Re-admission rates: an indicator of the quality of care' *BJHC* , Vol.6. No.10, pp.12-13.

Greer, A. L. (1977) 'Advances in the study of diffusion and innovation in health care organizations', *Milbank Quarterly*, Vol.55, pp.505-32.

________. (1981) 'Medical technology: assessment, adoption and utilization', *Journal of Medical Systems*, Vol.5, No.1/2, pp.129-45.

Griffith's Report (1983) *NHS Management Inquiry* , London: HMSO.

Grint, K. (1991) *The Sociology of Work: an introduction*, Cambridge: Polity Press.
Gunton, T. (1990) *Dictionary of Information Technology and Computer Science*, Harmondsworth: Penguin.
Habermas, J. (1976) *Legitimation Crisis*, London: Heinemann.
Hall, S., Critcher, C., Jefferson, T., Clarke, J. and Roberts B.(1978) *Policing the Crisis* , London: Macmillan.
Ham, C. (1992) *Health Policy in Britain: the politics and organisation of the National Health Service* (Third edition), London: Macmillan.
Ham, C., Robinson, R. and Benzeval, M. (1990) *Health Check: Health care reforms in an international context*, London: King's Fund Institute.
Hammersley, M. and Atkinson, P.(1983) *Ethnography: principles in practice* , London: Tavistock.
________. (1995) *Ethnography: principles in practice* (second edition), London: Routledge.
Hanby, J. G. (1974) 'Successful design management of integrated terminal-based medical systems', in J. Anderson and J. M. Forsythe (eds) *MEDINFO 1974: Proceedings of the First World Conference on Medical Informatics, Stockholm, August 5-10*, Oxford: North-Holland, pp.79-83.
Harrison, S. and Schulz, R.I. (1989) 'Clinical autonomy in the UK and the USA: contrasts and convergence', in G. Freddi and J.W. Björkman (eds) *Controlling Medical Professions: the comparative politics of health governance.* Sage: London, pp.198-209.
Harrison, S. and Pollitt, C. (1994) *Controlling Health Professionals*, Buckingham: Open University Press.
Harvey, D. (1989) *The Condition of Postmodernity,* Oxford: Blackwell.
Hassard, J. (1990) 'An alternative to paradigm incommensurability in organization theory', in J. Hassard and D. Pym (eds) *The Theory and Philosophy of Organizations*, London: Routledge, pp.219-230.
________. (1992) 'Multiple paradigms and organizational analysis: a case study', *Organization Studies*, Vol.12, No.2, pp.275-99.
________. (1993) 'Postmodernism and organizational analysis: an overview', in J. Hassard and M. Parker (eds) *Postmodernism and Organizations*, London: Sage, pp.1-24.
Hassard, J. and Pym, D. (eds) (1990) *The Theory and Philosophy of Organizations*, London: Routledge.
Hassard, J and Parker, M. (eds) (1993)*Postmodernism and Organizations* London: Sage.
Hausam, R.R. and Balas, A. (1993) 'Computerized medical records: dream or reality?' *Missouri Medicine, Vol.90*, No.10, pp.649-52.
Heath, C. (1982) 'Preserving the consultation: medical record cards and professional conduct', *Sociology of Health and Illness*, Vol.4, No.1, pp.56-74.
Henderson, J., Goldacre, M. J., Graveney, M. J. and Simmons, H.M. (1989) 'Use of medical record linkage to study re-admission rates' *British Medical Journal* , 16th September, pp.709-13.

Herring, J.E. (1991) 'Information management - the convergence of professions', *International Journal of Information Management*, Vol.11, pp.144-55.

Heydebrand, W.V. (1989) 'New organizational forms', *Work and Occupations,* Vol.16, No.3, pp.323-57.

Hills, J. (1984) *Information Technology and Industrial Policy*, Beckenham: Croom Helm.

Hindness, B. (1988) *Choice, Rationality and Social Theory*, London: Unwin Hyman.

HMSO (1989a) *Working for Patients* (CM 555), London.

HMSO (1989b) 'Medical audit', *NHS Review, Working Paper, No 6*, London.

Hochschild, A.R. (1983) *The Managed Heart: Commercialisation of Human Feeling*, London: University of California Press.

Hodson, R. and Parker, R.E. (1988) 'Work in high-technology settings: a review of the empirical literature.' *Research in the Sociology of Work* Vol.4, pp.1-29.

Holoien, M. O. (1977)*Computers and their Societal Impact*, London: Wiley.

Home Office (1978) *Report of the Committee on Data Protection* (Chairperson: Sir Norman Lindop) Cmnd.7341, London: HMSO.

Hsu, J. and Kusnan, J. (1989) *The Fifth Generation: the future of computer technology*, Blue Ridge Summit, PA: Windcrest Books.

Hughes, T.P.(1986) 'The seamless web: technology, science, etcetara, etcetera' *Social Studies of Science* , Vol.16, pp.281-92.

________. (1987) ' The evolution of large technological systems', in W.E. Bijker, T.P.Hughes, and T.J. Pinch, (eds) (1987) *The Social Construction of Technological Systems* MIT Press: London, pp.51-82.

Illsley, R.(1980) *Professional or Public Health?* London: NPHT.

Jahoda, M. (1989) 'Artificial intelligence: an outsider's perspective', in Forester, T. (ed.) *Computers in the Human Context: information technology and people*. Oxford: Blackwell, pp.144-56

James, N. (1988) 'Care = Organisation + Physical labour + Emotional Labour', *Paper presented at the BSA Medical Sociology Conference*, University of York.

Jamous, H. and Peloille, B. (1970) 'Professions or self-perpetrating systems? Changes in the French university-hospital system', in J.A. Jackson (ed.) *Professions and Professionalization*, Cambridge: Cambridge University Press, pp.109-152.

Jaques, E. (1951) *The Changing Culture of a Factory*, London: Tavistock.

Jaques, E. with members of the Brunel Health Services Organisation Research Unit (1978) *Health Services: their nature and organisation, and role of patients, doctors, nurses and the complementary professions*, London: Heinemann.

Jessop, B. Bonnett, K. and Ling, T. (1988) *Thatcherism* , Cambridge: Polity Press.

Johnson, T. (1972) *Professions and Power, London*: Macmillan.

________. (1976) 'The professions in the class structure', in R. Scase (ed.) *Industrial Society: class, cleavage and control*, London: Allen & Unwin, pp.93-110.

________. (1982) 'The state and the professions: peculiarities of the British', in A. Giddens and G. Mackenzie (eds) *Social Class and the Division of Labour*, Cambridge: Cambridge University Press, pp.186-208.

________. (1995) 'Governmentality and the institutionalization of expertise', in T. Johnson, G. Larkin, and M. Saks, M. (eds) *Health Professions in Europe*. London: Routledge, pp.7-24.

Johnson, T. Larkin, G. and Saks, M. (eds) (1995) *Health Professions in Europe*. London: Routledge.

Jones, B.T. (1991) 'Building nursing expert systems: using automated rule induction.' *Computers in Nursing,* Vol 9, No.2, pp.52-60.

Kaplan, B. (1982) 'User acceptance of medical computer applications: a diffusion approach', in B.I. Blum (ed.) *Proceedings of the 6th Conference on Computers in Health Care.* Long Beach, California: IEEE Computer Publications.

Kearsley, N., Little, T. and Wiseman, C. (1994) 'Realised potential' *Nursing Times.* Vol.90, No.24, (15 June), pp.44-5.

Keen, J. (1994) 'Information Policy in the National Health Service', in J. Keen (ed.) *Information Management in Health Services.* Buckingham: Open University Press, pp.16-28.

________. (1994) 'Evaluation: informing the future, not living in the past', in J. Keen (ed.) *Information Management in Health Services.* Buckingham: Open University Press, pp.171-83.

Keen, J. and Malby, R. (1992) 'Nursing power and practice in the United Kingdom National Health Service.' *Journal of Advanced Nursing*, Vol.17, pp.863-70.

Kenny, D.J. (1974) 'Management tactics for the introduction of computers into health care units', in J. Anderson and J.M. Forsythe (eds) *MEDINFO 74: proceedings of the first world conference on medical informatics, Stockholm, August 5-10*, Oxford: North-Holland, pp.127-31

Kerrison, S. (1993) 'Contracting and the quality of medical care', in I. Tilley (ed.) *Managing the Internal Market*, London: Paul Chapman, pp.138-145.

Kerrison, S., Packwood, T. and M. Buxton (1993) *Medical Audit: taking stock*, Medical Audit Series No.6: Kings' Fund Centre: London.

Klein, R. (1989) *The Politics of the National Health Service* (second edition), London: Longman.

Knights, D. (1990) 'Subjectivity, power and the labour process', in D. Knights and H. Willmott (eds) *Labour Process Theory*, London: Macmillan, pp.297-335.

Knights, D. and Willmott, H. (1990) 'Introduction', in D. Knights, and H. Willmott, (eds) *Labour Process Theory*, London: Macmillan,. pp.1-45.

Knights, D. and Vurdubakis, T. (1994) 'Foucault, power, resistance and all that' in J.M. Jermier, D. Knights and W.R. Nord (eds) *Resistance and Power in Organizations*, London: Routledge, pp.167-98.

Kraft, P.(1979) 'The industrialization of computer programming: from programming to "software production"', in A. Zimbalist (ed.) *Case Studies on the Labor Process* London: Monthly Review Press, pp.1-17

Krause, E. (1977) *Power and Illness*, New York: Elsevier.

Lamb, G. M. (1973) *Computers in the Public Service*, London: Allen & Unwin.

Larson, M. S. (1977) *The Rise of Professionalism: a sociological analysis*, London: University of California Press.

________. (1980) 'Proletarianization and educated labor', *Theory and Society*, Vol.9, No.1, pp.131-75.

Lash, S. (1990) *The Sociology of Postmodernism,* London: Routledge.

Lash, S. and Urry, J. (1984) 'The new Marxism of collective action' *Sociology,* Vol 18, No 1, pp.32-50.

________. (1987) *The End of Organized Capitalism,* Cambridge: Polity Press

________. (1994) *Economies of Signs and Space*, London: Sage.

Latour, B. (1987) *Science in Action.*, Milton Keynes: Open University Press.

________. (1988) '*The Prince* for machines as well as machinations', in B. Elliott (ed.), *Technology and Social Process*, Edinburgh: Edinburgh University Press, pp.20-43.

________. (1993) *We Have Never Been Modern*, Hemel Hempstead: Harvester Wheatsheaf.

Laurance, J. (1981) 'Why the DHSS computer advisers resigned' *Medical World*, Vol.16, No.12, 12th March, pp.23-6.

Law, J. (ed.) (1991) *A Sociology of Monsters: essays on power, technology and domination*, London: Routledge.

________. (1992) 'Notes on the theory of the actor-network: ordering, strategy, and heterogeneity', *Systems Practice*, Vol.5, No.4, pp.379-93.

Leavitt, H.J. and Whisler, T.L. (1958) 'Management in the 1980s' *Harvard Business Review,* 36, No.6, pp.41-8.

Lévi-Strauss, C. (1966) *The Savage Mind*, London: Weidenfeld and Nicolson.

Lindberg, D.A.B. (1979) 'The development and diffusion of medical technology: medical information systems' Appendix E. *A Report by the Committee on Technology and Health Care.* Washington D.C: National Academy of Sciences.

Lockwood, D. (1958) *The Blackcoated Worker*, London: Allen & Unwin

Lyons, D. (1988) *The Information Society: issues and illusions* Cambridge: Polity Press.

McCormick, K.A. (1986) 'Research applications' (Chapter 14), in V.K. Saba and K.A. McCormick (eds) *Essentials of Computers for Nurses,* Philadelphia and London: Lippincott, pp.330-61.

McColl, I., Fernow, L. C., Mackie, C., and Rendall, M. (1976) 'Communication as a method of medical audit', *The Lancet* (19th June), pp.1342-4.
McIntyre, N. Day, R.C. and Pearson, A.J.G. (1972) 'Can we write better notes? An introduction to Problem Orientated Medical Records (the Weed approach),' *British Journal of Hospital Medicine* (May), pp.603-11.
MacIntyre, S. (1976) 'Some notes on record taking and making in an antenatal clinic', *Sociological Review*, Vol.26, No.13, pp.595-611.
Mackenzie, D. and Wajcman, J. (eds) (1985) *The Social Shaping of Technology*, Milton Keynes: Open University Press.
McKinlay, J. and Arches, J. (1985) 'Towards the proletarianization of physicians' *International Journal of Health Services, Vol.15*, pp.161-95.
McLaughlin, K., Taylor, S., Bliss-Holtz, J., Saayers, P.and Nickle, L. (1990) 'Shaping the future: the marriage of nursing theory and informatics.' *Computers in Nursing* Vol.8, No.4, pp.174-9.
McLoughlin, I. and Clark, J. (1994) *Technology and Change at Work* (second edition), Buckingham: Open University Press.
McSherry, C.K. (1976) 'Quality assurance: the cost of utilization review and the educational value of medical audit in a university hospital' *Surgery*, Vol.80, No.1, pp.122-9.
Malby, R. and Clayton, J. (1994) 'Nursing information', in J. Keen (ed) *Information Management in Health Services*, Buckingham: Open University Press, pp.74-87.
Marmor, T.R. and Plowden, W.(1991) 'Spreading the sickness' *Times Higher Educational Supplement,* 17, 25th October , p.17.
Mason, A. (1984) 'Körner progress report' *BJHC*, Vol.1, No.1, pp.24-5.
Merrison, A. W. (Chairperson) (1979) *Royal Commission on the NHS*, London: HMSO.
Michie, D. and Johnston, R. (1985) *The Creative Computer: machine intelligence and human knowledge*, Harmondsworth: Penguin.
The Milbank Quarterly (1988) *The Changing Character of the Medical Profession* , Vol.66, Supplement 2.
Miller, R.A. Pople, H.E. and Myers, J. (1984) 'INTERNIST-1, an experimental computer-based diagnostic consultant for general internal medicine', In W.J. Clancey and Shortliffe, E.H. (eds) *Readings in Medical Artificial Intelligence,* London: Addison-Wesley, pp.190-209.
Millman, M. (1977) *The Unkindest Cut*, New York: Morrow & Co.
Morgan, G. (1986) *Images of Organizations*, London: Sage.
Moritz, P.(1990) 'Information technology: a priority for nursing research.' *Computers in Nursing*, Vol.8, No.3, pp.111-15.
Mountney, L. and Sanderson, H. (1993) 'The long and short of it', *Health Services Journal*, 9 December, pp.36-7.
Mumford, E. and Banks, O. (1967) *The Computer and the Clerk*, London: Routledge and Kegan Paul .

Murray, F. and Knights, D. (1990) 'Inter-managerial competition and capital accumulation: IT specialists, accountants and executive control', *Critical Perspectives on Accounting,* Vol.1, No.2, pp.167-89.

National Audit Office (NAO) (1988) *Quality of Clinical Care in Hospitals,* London: HMSO.

________. (1990) *Managing computer projects in the NHS*, London: HMSO.

NHS/DHSS (Chairperson: Mrs E. Körner) (1982a) *The First Report: the collection and use of information about clinical activity*, London: HMSO.

NHS/DHSS (Chairperson: Mrs E. Körner) (1982b) *The Third Report: the collection and use of information about health service manpower*, London: HMSO.

________. (1984) *The Sixth Report: the collection and use of information about health service finance*, London: HMSO.

NHS/Department of Health (1990) *National Health Service Review: working for patients: framework for information systems: information technology* (Project 25), Elephant and Castle, London: Information Management Group (IMG).

NHS Management Executive (1993) *Clinical audit in HCHS: allocation of funds 1993/94. Circular EL (93) 34*, Department of Health: Leeds

________. (1994) *Clinical audit :1994/95 and beyond. Circular EL (94 20,* Department of Health: Leeds

Newman, M. and Rosenberg, D. (1985) 'Systems analysts and the politics of organizational control', *Omega*, Vol.13, No.5, pp.393-406.

Ngin, P.Simms, L.M. and Erbin-Roesemann (1993) 'Work excitement among computer users in nursing.' *Computers in Nursing* Vol.11, No.3. pp.127-33.

Noble, D. F. (1979) 'Social choice in machine design: the case of automatically controlled machine tools', in A. Zimbalist (ed.) *Case Studies on the Labor Process*, New York: Monthly Review Press, pp.18-50.

Noble, D. F. (1985) 'Social choice in machine design: the case of automatically controlled machine tools', in D. MacKenzie and J. Wacjman (eds) *The Social Shaping of Technology* Milton Keynes: Open University Press, pp.109-24.

Nolan, R. (1979) 'Managing the crisis in data processing'. *Harvard Business Review,* Vol.57, No.2, pp.115-26.

O'Connor, J. (1973) *The Fiscal Crises of the State*, New York: St Martin's Press.

________. (1984) *Accumulation Crisis*, Oxford: Blackwell.

O'Dell, D.V., Tape, T.G. and Campbell, J.R. (1992) 'Increasing physician acceptance and use of the computerized ambulatory medical record'. *Proceedings - the Annual Symposium on Computer Applications in Medical Care*. Long Beach, California: IEEE Computer Society Press, pp.848-52.

O'Neil, M. (1993) 'Read all about it', *BJHC*, Vol.10, No.10, pp.22-3.

Offe, C. and Wiesenthal, H. (1980) 'Two logics of collective action: theoretical notes on social class and organizational form, *Political Power and Social Theory, 1* edited by M. Zeitlin Greenwich: Jai, pp.67-115
Olson, M. (1965) *The Logic of Collective Action*, Cambridge, Mass: Harvard University Press.
Opit, L.J. and Woodroffe, F.J. (1970) 'Computer held clinical record system-II assessment' *British Medical Journal*, Vol.4, 10th October, pp.80-2.
Oppenheimer, M. (1973) 'The proletarianization of the professional', *Sociological Review Monograph*, No. 20.
Orchard, C. (1994) 'Comparing healthcare outcomes'. *British Medical Journal*, Vol.308, pp.1493-6. .
Ouchi, W.G. (1991) 'Markets, bureaucracies and clans', in G. Thompson, J. Frances, R. Levacic and J. Mitchell (eds) *Markets, Hierarchies and Networks: the coordination of social life*, London: Sage, pp.246-55.
Packwood, T., Keen, J. and Buxton, M. (1991) *Hospitals in Transition: The Resource Management Initiative,* Milton Keynes: Open University Press.
Packwood, T., Kerrison, S. and Buxton, M. (1994) 'The implementation of medical audit'. *Social Policy and Administration* ,Vol.28, No.4, pp.299-316.
Pahl, R.E. and Winkler, J.T. (1974) 'The economic elite: theory and practice', in P.Stanworth and A. Giddens (eds) *Elites and Power in British Society*, Cambridge: Cambridge University Press, pp.102-22.
Parker, M. (1992) 'Post-modern organizations or postmodern organization theory?' *Organization Studies,* Vol.13, No.1, pp.1-17.
________. (1993) 'Life after Jean-François', in J. Hassard and M. Parker (eds) *Postmodernism and Organizations*, London: Sage, pp.204-12.
Paul, R. (1995) 'Burton: a self-funding HISS achieving success through staff commitment', *BJHC*, Vol.12, No.10, pp.32-3.
Peel, V, Nicholson, L. and Walker, H. (1994) 'An inspector calls'. *Health Services Management*, June, pp.14-17.
Peters, T. J. and Waterman, R. H. (1982) *In Search of Excellence*, New York: Harper and Row.
Pettigrew, A. M. (1972) 'Information control as a power resource', *Sociology*, Vol.6, No.2, pp.187-204.
________. (1973a) *The Politics of Organizational Decisionmaking*, London: Tavistock.
________. (1973b) 'Occupational specialization as an emergent process'. *The Sociological Review* ,Vol 21, No 2, pp.255-78.
________. (1974) 'The influence process between specialists and executives', *Personnel Review*, Vol.3, No.1, pp.24-30.
________. (1975) 'Strategic aspects of the management of specialist activity', *Personnel Review*, Vol.4, No.1, pp.5-13.
________. (1985) *The Awakening Giant: continuity and change in ICI*, Oxford: Blackwell.
Pinch, T.J. and Bijker, W.E. (1984) 'The social construction of facts and artefacts', *Social Studies of Science*, Vol.14, pp.399-441.

________. (1987) 'The social construction of facts and artefacts: or how the sociology of science and the sociology of technology might benefit each other', in W. E. Bijker, T. P.Hughes, and T. J. Pinch (eds)*The Social Construction of Technological Systems* , MIT Press: London, pp.17-50.

Piore and Sabel (1984) *The Second Industrial Divide* New York, Basic Books.

Powell, W. W. (1991) 'Neither market nor hierarchy' in Thompson, G., Frances, J., Levacic and Mitchell, J. (eds) *Markets, Hierarchies and Networks: the coordination of social life*, London: Sage. pp.256-76.

Preston, A. Cooper, D. and Coombs, R. (1989) 'Fabricating budgets: a case study of the production of management budgeting in the National Health Service' Unpublished Paper, November, 1989.

Public Accounts Commission (PAC) (1989) *Quality of Clinical Care in NHS Hospitals,* London: HMSO.

Rabinow, P.(ed.) (1984) *The Foucault Reader* London: Penguin.

Ranade, W. (1994) *A Future for the NHS? Health care in the 1990s.* London: Longman.

Read, S.M. and George, S. (1994) 'Nurse practitioners in A & E departments: reflections on a pilot study' *Journal of Advanced Nursing*, Vol.19, No.4 (April), pp.105-16.

Rector, A. L., Kay, S. and Howkins, T.J. 'A human computer interface for doctors', in P.Starling with J Guinnane (eds) *Pulling Together: current perspectives in health computing,* The British Computer Society Health Informatics Specialist Group-The BJHC: Weybridge, pp 213-22.

Reed, M.I. (1992) *The Sociology of Organizations: themes, perspectives and prospects,* London: Harvester-Wheatsheaf.

Rees, C. (1981) 'Records and hospital routine', in P.Atkinson, and C. Heath (eds) *Medical Work: realities and routines.* Aldershot: Gower, pp.55-70.

Reiser, S.J. (1978) *Medicine and the Reign of Technology*, Cambridge: Cambridge University Press.

Resource Management Directorate (1989) *Information Package-Acute Hospitals: the six experimental sites* , London: Department of Health.

Richman, J. (1987) *Medicine and Health*, London, Longman.

Riesbeck, C. and Schank, R. (1989) *Inside Case Based Reasoning.* Hillside, New Jersey: Lawrence Erlbaum Associates.

Riley, J.B. (1996) 'Educational applications', in V.K. Saba and K.A. McCormick (eds) *Essentials of Computers for Nurses* (second edition), Philadelphia and London: Lippincott Company, PP. 528-573.

Rios, H., Delaney, C., Kruckeberg, T. Chung, Y. and Mehmert, P.A.(1991) 'Validation of defining characteristics of four nursing diagnosis using a computerized data-base' *Journal of Professional Nursing*, Vol.5, No.5, pp.293-9.

Ritzer, G. (1993) *The McDonaldization of Society*. Thousands Oaks, California: Pine Forge Press.

Robinson, R. (1994) 'Hospitals in the market', in J. Keen (ed.) *Information Management in Health Services.* Buckingham: Open University Press, pp.3-15.

Roemer, M. I. and Friedman, J.W. (1971) *Doctors in Hospitals*, Baltimore: John Hopkins Press.

Rogers, E.M. (1962) *Diffusion of Innovation*, New York: Free Press.

________. (1971) *Communication of Innovation: a cross cultural approach* (second edition), New York: Free Press. .

Rose, H. (1991) 'The emergent IT-based enterprise?', in *New Technology and Manufacturing: the UK experience* (TORU Occasional Paper No.3), M. Dent and M. Parker (eds) Stoke on Trent: Staffordshire University, School of Social Sciences, pp.95-105.

Rowbottom, R. (1977) *Social Analysis: a collaborative method of gaining usable scientific knowledge of social institutions*, London: Heinemann.

Royal College of Physicians (1989) *Medical Audit: A first report. What, why and how?* London: The Royal College of Physicians of London.

Rundell, S. (1991) 'Are you obsessed with IT? *Nursing Times* Vol.87, No.41, October, 9. p.24.

Rustin, M. (1989) 'The politics of post-Fordism or trouble with the "New Times"', *New Left Review*, 21, July: 55-77.

Rustin, M. (1995) 'The idea of community and the non-profit sector', *Renewal*, Vol.3, No.2, pp.25-34.

Saba, V. K. and McCormick, K. A. (eds) (1986) *Essentials of Computers for Nurses,* Philadelphia and London: Lippincott Company.

________. (1996) *Essentials of Computers for Nurses* (second edition), Philadelphia and London: Lippincott Company.

Sacks, H., Schegloff, E. and Jefferson, G. (1974) 'A simplest systematics for the analysis of turn-taking for conversation'. *Language*, Vol.50, pp.696-735.

Sakolsky, R. (1992) '"Disciplinary power" and the labour process', in A. Sturdy, D. Knights and H. Willmott (eds) *Skill and Consent: contemporary studies in the labour process,* London: Routledge, pp.235-54.

Salvage, J. (1989) 'The double-edged sword.' *Nursing Times*, Vol.85, No.5, 1989, pp.64-5.

Sanazaro, P.J. (1974) 'Medical audit: experience in the USA', *British Medical Journal* , 16th February, pp.271-4.

Scheff, T.J. (1978) 'Decisions in medicine', in P.Worsley (ed.) *Problems of Modern Society* (second edition), Harmondsworth: Penguin, pp.607-14.

Schieber, G.J., Poullier, J-P.and Greenwald, L. (1992) 'US health expenditure performance: an international comparison and data update', *Health Care Financing Review*, Vol.13, No.4, pp.1-87.

Schneiderman, B. (1987) *Designing the User Interface: strategies for effective human-computer interaction*, Reading, Mass.: Addison-Wesley.

Scrivens, E. (1985) *Policy, Power and Information Technology in the National Health Service*. Bath Social Policy Papers, University of Bath.
Scrivens, E.(1988) 'The management of clinicians in the NHS' *Social Policy and Administration* , Vol.22, No.1, pp.22-34.
Secretary of State for Health and Others (1989) *Working for Patients*, London: HMSO.
Sewell, G. and Wilkinson, B. (1992) '"Someone to watch over me": surveillance, discipline, and the just-in-time labour process', *Sociology* Vol.26, No.2, pp.271-90.
Sharples, S. (1987) 'DRGs and computing' *BJHC*, Vol.4., No.5, pp 27-31.
Shaw, C. D. (1980a) 'Aspects of audit: 1. The background' *British Medical Journal*, 24 May, pp.1256-8.
Shaw, C. D. (1980b) 'Aspects of audit: 5. looking forward to audit' *British Medical Journal*, 21 June. pp.1509-11.
Shaw, C. D. and Costain, D.W. (1989) 'Guide-lines for medical audit: seven principles' *British Medical Journal*, Vol.299, pp.498-9.
Sheil, B. (1989) 'Thinking about artificial intelligence', in Forester, T. (ed.) *Computers in the Human Context: Information Technology and People*. Oxford: Blackwell, pp.157-73.
Shortliffe, E. H. (1976) *Computer-Based Medical Consultations: MYCIN*, Oxford: Elsevier/North-Holland.
________. (1983) 'Medical consultation systems: designing for doctors', in M. E. Sime and M. J. Coombs (eds) *Designing for human-computer communications*, London: Academic Press, pp.209-38.
________. (1984) 'Knowledge engineering for medical decision making: a review of computer-based clinical decision aids', in W.J. Clancey and E.H. Shortliffe (eds) *Readings in Medical Artificial Intelligence: the first decade*. London: Addison-Wesley, pp.35-71.
________. (1986) 'Computer-based medical consultation systems' *The Stanford Computer Science Video Journal: AI Research Lectures*. San Mateo, Calif.: Morgan Kauffman.
Shortliffe, E. H., Davis, R., Axline, S. G., Buchanan, B. G., Green, C. C., and Cohen, N. (1975) 'Computer-based consultations in clinical therapeutics: explanation and rule-acquisition capabilities of the MYCIN system'. *Computer and Biomedical Research*. Vol.8., No.4, pp.303-20.
Shortliffe, E.H. and Perreault, L.E. (eds) (1990) *Medical Informatics: computer applications in health care*, Reading, Mass.: Addison-Wesley.
Silverman, D. (1970) *The Theory of Organizations*, London: Heinemann Educational Books.
________. (1985) *Qualitative Methodology & Sociology*, Aldershot: Gower.
________. (1994) 'On throwing away ladders: re-writing the theory of organizations', in J. Hassard and M. Parker (eds) *Towards a New Theory of Organizations*, London: Routledge, pp.1-23.
Smallman, A. (1992) 'Improving the image of medical records', *BJHC*, Vol.9, No.7, pp.18-20.

Smart, B. (1992) *Modern Conditions, Postmodern Controversies*, London: Routledge.
Smith, C. (1987) *Technical Workers: class, labour and trade unionism*, London: Macmillan.
Smith, M. (1994) 'IT futures in the NHS', in J. Keen (ed.) *Information Management in Health Service*, Buckingham: Open University Press, pp.184-98.
Smith, M.C. and Hutchinson, E.C. (1975) 'Introduction', in Staffordshire Area Health Authority *Computers in Health Care: papers given at a symposium on real-time computer systems implemented in the North Staffordshire Hospital Centre*, Stoke on Trent: Staffordshire AHA (North Staffordshire District), pp.1-9.
Sorenson, L. (1991) *Nursing and Computers: caring in the context of information technology*, Unpublished Ph.D. City University of New York, USA.
Stacey, M. (1981) 'The division of labour revisited or overcoming the two Adams', in P.Abrams, R. Deem, J. Finch and P.Rock (eds) *Practice and Progress: British sociology 1950-80*, London: George Allen & Unwin.
Starkey, K. (1992) 'Time and the consultant: issues of contract and control', in R. Loveridge and K. Starkey (eds) *Continuity and Crisis in the NHS* , Buckingham: Open University Press, pp.54-64
Stokes, A. (1988a) 'Computers linking computers' *BJHC*, Vol.5, No.3, pp.32-5.
________. (1988b) 'NHS data communications and international standards', in Starling, P (sub ed.) with Guinnane, J. *Current Perspectives in Health Computing: conference and exhibition, Brighton Metropole. 9-11 May*, Weybridge: BJHC, pp.140-3.
________. (1989) 'Patient data transfer by OSI' *BJHC*, Vol.6, No.1 (February), pp.33-5.
Strauss, A. Fagerhaugh, S. Suczec, B. and Wiener, C. (1982) 'Sentimental work in the technologized hospital', *Sociology of Health and Illness*, Vol.4, No.3, pp.254-78.
________. (1985) *Social Organization of Medical Work*.. London: University of Chicago Press.
Strong, P.(1979) *The Ceremonial Order of the Clinic* London: Routledge and Kegan Paul.
________. (1982) 'Power, etiquette and identity in medical consultation'. *Paper presented at the BSA. Annual Conference, University of Durham*..
Szolovits, P.(1982) 'Artificial intelligence in medicine', in P.Szolovits (ed.) *Artificial Intelligence in Medicine*, Boulder, Colorado: Westview Press for the American Association of the Advancement of Science, pp.1-19.
Taylor, T.R. (1980) 'The role of computer systems in medical decision-making', in H. T. Smith and T. R. G. Green (eds) *Human Interaction With Computers*, London: Academic Press, pp.231-66.
The Times, (1982) 'A case history of a fading hospital dream', London, 5th October, p.13.

Thompson, J. B. (1984) *Studies in the Theory of Ideology*, Cambridge, Polity Press.

Thompson, P.(1990) 'Crawling from the wreckage: the labour process and the politics of production', in D. Knights and H. Willmott (eds) *Labour Process Theory*, London: Macmillan, pp.95-124.

________. (1993) 'Post-modernism: fatal distraction', in J. Hassard and M. Parker (eds) *Postmodernism and Organizations*, London: Sage, pp.304-42.

Tolliday, H. (1978) 'Clinical autonomy', in E. Jaques and members of the Brunel Health Services Organisation Research Unit (eds) *Health Services*, London: Heinemann, pp.32-52.

Troll, S. (1995) 'Computerising the clinical record', *BJHC,* Vol.12, No.8, pp.37-40.

Tuckman, A. and Blackburn, D. (1991) 'Fitness for purpose: total quality management in the health service'. *Paper presented at the Annual Conference of the British Sociological Association, Manchester.*

Turner, B.S. (1987) *Medical Power and Social Knowledge*, London: Sage.

Urry, J. (1990) *The Tourist Gaze*. London: Sage.

Vliet, H. (1993) *Software Engineering,* Chichester: Wiley.

Wacjman, J. (1991) *Feminism Confronts Technology*, Cambridge: Polity.

Waitzkin, H. and Stoeckle, J.D. (1976) 'Information control and the micropolitics of health care: summary of an ongoing research project', *Social Science and Medicine*, Vol.10, pp.263-76.

Walby, S. and Greenwell, J. with Mackay, L. and Soothill, K. (1994) *Medicine and Nursing: professions in a changing health service*, London: Sage.

Walker, M.B. (1986) 'Nursing education: challenges of the computerized environment.' *Computers in Nursing* Vol 4, No.4, pp.166-71.

Walton, I. (1986) *The Nursing Process in Perspective: a literature review*, Department of Social Policy and Social Work, University of York/DHSS.

Wardle, A. and Wardle, L. (1978) 'Computer-aided diagnosis - a review of research', *Methods of Information in Medicine,* Vol.17, No.1, pp.15-28.

Warren, L. (1992) 'Power, corruption and lies', *BJHC*, Vol.9, No.7, pp.9-12.

Waters, M. (1994) *Modern Sociological Theory*, London: Sage.

Webster, F. (1995) *Theories of The Information Society*, London: Routledge.

Weed, L.L. (1968) 'Medical records that guide and teach' *New England Journal of Medicine* Vol.278, No.12, pp.593-600 and 652-7.

________. (1969) *Medical Records, Medical Education and Patient Care*, Cleveland: The Press of the Case Western Reserve University.

Weinberg, N. (1990) *Computers in the Information Society*, Boulder, San Francisco and Oxford: Westview Press.

Weizenbaum, J. (1984) *Computer Power and Human Reason: from judgement to calculation*. Harmondsworth: Penguin Books.

West Midlands RHA (1979) *WMRHA MUMPS Project at Walsall: evaluation document for the DHSS*, Birmingham: Management Services Division.
Westin, A.F. (1976) *Computers, Health Records and Citizen Rights*, Washington: National Bureau of Standards, Monograph 157: US Printing Office.
Wilkinson, B. (1983) *The Shopfloor Politics of New Technology*, London: Heinemann Educational Books.
Will, E.J. and Selwood, N.H. (1985) 'Computerised information for renal medicine', *BJHC*, Vol.2, No.1, pp 11-18.
Willcocks, L. and Mason, D. (1987) *Computerising Work*, London: Paradigm.
Williams, A.J., Smith, B.A., and Walls, J. (1984) 'End stage renal failure: coping with the demand', *Health Trends*, Vol.16 No.1 pp.1-3
Williamson, O. E. (1975) *Markets and Hierarchies: analysis and antitrust implications,* New York: Free Press.
Willis, J. (1994) 'Program for change' *Health Services Journal*, 26 May, pp.13-14.
Witz, A. (1992) *Professions and Patriarchy*, London: Routledge.
Wood, B. (1991) 'The non-achievement of cost containment in American health care: explanations and lessons for Britain'. *Public Policy and Administration*, Vol.6, No.3, pp.22-39.
Yang, T.F., Devine, B., and McFarlane, P.W. (1993) 'Deterministic logic versus software artificial neural networks in the diagnosis of atrial fibrillation', *Journal of Electrocardiology,* Vol.26 (Supplement), pp.90-4.
Young, D. W. (1980) 'House officer information system - HOIS', *International Journal of Bio-Medical Computing*, Vol.11, pp.521-9.
________. (1982) 'A survey of decision aids for clinicians', *British Medical Journal*, Vol.285 pp.1332-6
________. (1984) 'What makes doctors use computers?', *Journal of the Royal Society of Medicine*, Vol.77, pp.663-7.
________. (1985) 'COSTAR and its medical query language', in J.R. Bryant and B. Kostrewski (eds) *Current Perspectives in Health Computing,* Weybridge: BJHC, pp.38-45.
Young, D, Chapman, T. and Poile, C. (1990) 'Physician reveal thyself' *The BJHC* Vol.7, No.9, pp.16-21.

Index